Two Wines:

A PROPER
UNDERSTANDING OF
"WINE" IN THE BIBLE

Two Wines:

A Proper Understanding of "Wine" in the Bible

RICHARD TEACHOUT

XULON PRESS

Xulon Press
2301 Lucien Way #415
Maitland, FL 32751
407.339.4217
www.xulonpress.com

Major revision and updating of
Grape Juice in the Bible: God's Blessing for His People
By the same author © 2011, Richard Teachout.

Unless otherwise indicated, Scripture quotations taken from the King
James Version (KJV) – *public domain.*

Printed in the United States of America.

ISBN-13: 978-1-6305-0110-5

These were more noble than those in Thessalonica, in that they received the word with all readiness of mind, and searched the scriptures daily, whether those things were so. (Acts 17:11)

Prove all things; hold fast that which is good. (1 Th. 5:21)

To my late pastor father,
who taught me that
God always speaks the truth to us
and
that He always speaks consistently in His Revelation.

To my brother (pastor, teacher, and author),
who in modern times pioneered the scholarship which finds
God's teaching about the fruit of the vine in the Bible to
be consistent.

To my wife, Nancy, and my missionary son, Raymond, for their
help and encouragement, and without whom this project would
never have been completed

TABLE OF CONTENTS

PREFACE

This book is a freshly edited and rewritten version of the book *Grape Juice in the Bible: God's Blessing for His People*, originally published by the present author in 2011. It is written to further clarify the teachings in the Bible concerning fresh grape juice in Bible times and alcoholic beverages, both in Bible times and in modern society.

Why publish this book since the understanding it produces of these two subjects is contrary to that of the majority of Bible scholars today who promote *moderate drinking* for Christians?

First, there is a great deal of confusion among these scholars, with many advancing theories and "facts" that are not true and are not in accord with proper understanding of the Bible or with written historical records. We will discuss these erroneous teachings.

Second, in our time, more and more of the scientific community is publishing fresh reports of the danger of alcohol. In 1983, when my wife and I had been ministering in France for five years, there was a slight change in public news concerning alcohol and its effects. When we first arrived in France, we learned quickly the importance of the wine industry, both socially and economically. There was never mention in newspapers or television of alcohol as a cause for an accident and very few negative alcohol-related articles appeared at all. Then it started to change dramatically. I remember a bill-board campaign in 1988 which appeared all over France that had two pictures: one showed happy people, each with a glass of wine in front of them and the other showed a horrible picture of an automobile accident. The caption under the pictures was very clear: "Un verre, ca va. Deux verres-bonjour les degats!" This means in English, "One glass, that's good-two glasses, disaster!" Since that time, there is even more realization of the dangers of alcohol. Very recently, a French publication cited an article which gave the findings of a study by a reputable organization in the USA that concluded there were no safe levels of alcohol, declaring that there were three million deaths in 2016 (worldwide) attributed to alcohol and that alcoholic consumption brings with it "massive health risks." The published report was sensational. The author of the report, Joshua Gowin, PhD, starts by asking, "Is the conventional wisdom wrong about booze?"

No healthy level of alcohol says major study.
Government should consider advising people to abstain completely, says authors. [1]

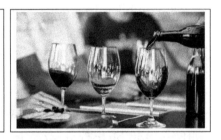

Here is an excerpt:

> A new scientific study concludes there is no safe level of drinking alcohol.
>
> The study, published in the inter-national medical journal, *The Lancet*, shows that in 2016, nearly three million deaths globally were attributed to alcohol use, including twelve percent of deaths in males between the ages of 15 and 49.
>
> "The health risks associated with alcohol are massive," said Dr. Emmanuela Gakidou of the Institute for Health Metrics and Evaluation at the University of Washington and the senior author of

the study. "Our findings are consistent with other recent research, which found clear and convincing correlations between drinking and premature death, cancer, and cardiovascular problems. Zero alcohol consumption minimizes the overall risk of health loss."

Just one more very recent and startling statistic before we continue. A website called the "Advisory Board" put out a daily briefing which studies the "stunning rise in alcohol deaths":

According to a recent analysis from the **Institute for Health Metrics and Evaluation** at the **University of Washington**, the number of alcohol-related deaths in the United States rose by 35% between 2007 and 2017. In comparison, the overall death rate in the United States rose by 24% over that time.[2]

Thirdly, not only is the scientific community getting very serious about the dangers of drinking *any* alcohol, but there is a recent, growing movement that speaks of the need to *stop* drinking alcohol in order to simply feel better and healthier and more alive. This is most popularly known as the "sober-curious movement". Recently it stimulated an article by Caitlin Gibson in the Washington Post, which was reproduced in the local Grand Rapids Press. The article starts out with this story:

The turning point came at an evening soiree in the middle of December, when Mai Trinh spotted a friend's luminous face amid a crowd of cocktail-quaffing partygoers.

"She stood out-she looked absolutely radiant," recalls Trinh, 44, a corporate wellness consultant and mom of three in Alexandria, Virginia. "So I asked her, 'What's your secret, what are you doing?'" Trinh's friend had decided to temporarily bail on booze, after signing up for an alcohol-free challenge through an online program.

It wasn't the first time Trinh, who considered herself an occasional social drinker, had heard of the burgeoning "sober-curious" movement, which touts the appeal of an alcohol-free lifestyle... Trinh rang in the New Year sober, and hasn't had a drink in the months since.[3]

The article goes on to give the background of this story:

For years, alcohol has steadily seeped into the social fabric of motherhood, with pitchers of mimosas at morning playdates, thermoses of "mommy juice" on the soccer field sidelines and Facebook feeds filled with stylized memes declaring it's not really drinking alone if your kids are home. Studies show that women-especially women in their 30s and 40s-are drinking more than ever before.[4]

When I went on-line to google "sober-curious", of which I had never heard, I found a large variety of "hits". One of these was "Shop Sober Curious on Amazon", which listed 16 books promoting a sober life-style, with titles ranging from "The Unexpected Joy of Being Sober: Discovering a happy, healthy, wealthy alcohol-free life" to "23 Minutes In Hell: One Man's Story About What He Saw, Heard, and Felt in That Place of Torment". We can characterize this entire movement and its growing literature as being very personal and simple "I stopped drinking alcohol and I feel happier and healthier; you need to stop too!" Interestingly, this message is the absolute contrary of all of the TV advertisement for alcohol "Drink our product and you will be joyful and happy"!

The message then, from the scientific community as to the danger of moderate drinking and from the Sober-Curious movement that moderate drinking is not necessary for happiness is very interesting in a day when more and more Christians are starting to drink moderately and are defending their actions from the Bible. This present study on "two wines" will show that God did bless the consumption of fresh grape juice in His Holy Word and not only did not bless the drinking of an alcoholic wine in the Bible, but clearly and specifically condemns it.

In our bibliography we present a long list of books that have been published, which develop the same thesis as the present book concerning fresh grape juice and alcoholic beverages in Bible times and the dangers of moderate drinking. The first one (chronologically) was written and published in 1855 called *Strong Drink Delusion, with Its Criminal and Ruinous Results Exposed* by George Marshall, a Canadian judge who did massive studies on the subject in the 1840s. In 1857, Eliphalet Nott wrote *Lectures on Temperance*. William Patton wrote *The Laws of Fermentation and the Wines of the Ancients* in 1871. After that, his book went out of print and there was very little activity until Robert Teachout (brother of the present author) wrote his doctoral thesis on the subject and then published *Wine the Biblical Imperative: Total Abstinence* in 1971. Many good books have been published since.

In light of these excellent studies, the reader might wonder, "Why another book?" Because there are several important subjects which are not at all treated elsewhere, that we will treat in the present book. We will discuss:

1. Episodes from the life of the author, which help explain not only the truth of his presentation of the fact that fresh grape juice *was* available in Bible times but also the fact that God does *not* condone alcoholic beverages for His people.

2. A presentation of the science of interpreting biblical words and concepts which clearly show that understanding the words from the Bible that are translated by *wine* in the English Bible do **not** mean **only** "alcoholic wine" but **can and do often** mean "fresh grape juice." This will include a discussion of *truth*—and a look at how most Bible scholars understood *wine* today as referring only to an alcoholic drink.

3. A survey of the historical development of the fiery opposition to God's blessing alcohol in the Bible and in society by Bible teachers and preachers between 1920 and 1935, which was largely responsible for Prohibition in America.

4. A personal desire to change the mind of at least one young Christian family who is considering moderate drinking of alcohol.

In order to come to the truth of this important matter, we will have to look extensively at what the Scriptures say, citing many verses. We will also show extensive research of other sources, citing many authors who have studied the subject.

INTRODUCTION

I preached a series of four messages in October 2010 on "Wine in the Bible." My purpose was to enlighten Christians to the truth that God never encourages His children to partake of an alcoholic beverage. The third message, "God Blesses Grape Juice in the Bible," became the most important in that series. In that message, contrary to almost all Bible expositors of our day, I show from the Word of God that grape juice did indeed exist in Bible times. At the conclusion I asked and answered the question, "Does it matter?" Does it matter whether God's people in Bible times had only alcoholic wine to drink or rather that they had a choice between that and natural grape juice with no alcoholic content?

I realized at that point just how much it mattered, for this is the key to the entire debate on whether or not Christians should drink alcohol. I decided to rewrite the book "On the Fruit of the Vine: In Defense of Biblical Consistency" that I had written earlier. I feel that the erroneous idea that grape juice is not mentioned in the Bible is the reason why conservative Christians "en masse" have so drastically changed their teaching on alcohol in the last fifty years.

The result of the aggressive promotion of this erroneous teaching is that there has been a major push in recent times to promote an interpretation of Scripture that would affirm that Jesus Himself created an alcoholic beverage in His first miracle and drank of it Himself. Since He did this, we can too! The result is a major shift in Christian thought-more and more are promoting or condoning a Christian's right to drink alcohol. One startling manifestation of this is detailed in the following article. After 68 years of teaching and practicing abstinence, a former fundamentalist Bible college has changed its policy on moderate drinking! Why?

Because they now interpret the Bible to say that God permitted and encouraged it! Their president asserted that alcohol abstinence is "biblically indefensible."

The same article goes on to name nine other Christian colleges which have taken the same position.[5] Other church leaders have gone even further. Mark Driscoll, who is pastor of the Seattle-area Mars Hill Church and president of the "Acts 29" group of churches, wrote in his book, *Radical Reformission*, that abstinence from alcohol is a sin.[6]

Though the modern message concerning alcohol has changed, the Bible has not changed its message. The Bible still affirms clearly that all Scripture is inspired of God and is profitable for His children (2 Tim. 3:16). It is an absolute truth, fundamental to the Christian faith that God has spoken to man by His Word.

Can this God lie or fail to communicate clearly with His creatures? Absolutely *not*. A. W. Tozer said that worship rises or falls with our concept of God: "If there is one terrible disease in the Church of Christ today, it is that we do not see God as great as He is. We're too familiar with God." I can further state here that our understanding of God's Word rises or falls with our concept of God. He is the great and wonderful creator God of the universe. He has spoken to man.

He says that in His Word 300 times! Amos 4:13 says, "For, lo, He that formeth the mountains, and createth the wind, and

THE GRAND RAPIDS PRESS

SATURDAY, NOVEMBER 21, 2009

'Thou shalt not drink' revoked

Cornerstone University ends 68-year-old ban on imbibing for faculty, staff

BY KYM REINSTADLER
THE GRAND RAPIDS PRESS

GRAND RAPIDS — Cornerstone University is lifting a ban on faculty and staff alcohol use that has stood since the institution was founded 68 years ago.

President Joe Stowell told Cornerstone's 279 employees at a staff meeting Friday that alcohol abstinence — a component of a lifestyle statement that had to be signed every year — is being dropped because a three-year internal study concluded it is "biblically indefensible."

"Given scripture's lack of a prohibition against use of alcohol in moderation, we are releasing our faculty and staff to discern what is best for them concerning its use in their personal lives," said Stowell, in his second year as the university's president.

The change doesn't apply to students, who remain banned from using alcohol.

Faculty and staff are being told to avoid using alcohol in any setting where students are present. Corner-

Joe Stowell

MORE
■ Cornerstone cuts staff.

---

xx

declareth unto man what is His thought ... The LORD, The God of hosts, is His name."

We must understand that God's Word *never* contradicts itself. So, how can God be inconsistent in His Revelation concerning alcoholic beverages? Can He say in His Word that they are both good and bad, as some would understand today?

At the present time, there are three popular positions in America concerning Christians and alcoholic beverages:

1. The conviction that only one "wine" is mentioned in the Bible (which is always fermented) and thus Christians have every right to drink moderately.
2. The conviction that only one "wine" is mentioned in the Bible (alcoholic), but there are Biblical and other reasons for Christians to abstain from alcohol.
3. The conviction that two distinct "wines" are mentioned in the Bible: fresh grape juice and alcoholic wine. God clearly blesses the first and condemns the second.

The first two positions are the subject of many articles, messages, and internet blogs. They both interpret God's Word in such a way that He blesses and condones the same substance, alcoholic wine. Proponents of both positions assert that grape juice is not found in the Bible and did not exist as a beverage in Bible times, because there was no way to preserve it. The third position is held by those who believe that abstinence is the best policy for Christians and they do have an answer to what they perceive as God's seeming inconsistency in blessing and condemning the drinking of "wine": there are two wines! Unfortunately, because of the overwhelming popularity of the first two positions, the subject of wine in the Bible is something which is rarely discussed in fundamentalist and conservative evangelical churches-even though many of these churches have written policies prohibiting the use of alcoholic beverages for their members.

The result is foreseeable and is being quickly realized. Something new is growing in American Christianity: tolerance (and often promotion) of the consumption of alcohol. The result is that the alcoholic beverage industry is entering into our Christian community like a camel, which, once his nose is thrust into the tent, soon follows with his body. This camel is very dangerous. This will be discussed later, but in the meantime consider this:

- ✓ Drug experts say alcohol is worse than crack or heroin.[7]
- ✓ Study: Alcohol "most harmful drug," followed by crack and heroin.[8]
- ✓ LONDON-Alcohol is more dangerous than illegal drugs like heroin and crack cocaine, according to a new study.[9]
- ✓ Alcohol-related deaths account for almost 100,000 deaths per year in US.[10]
- ✓ WHO Reports that Alcohol-Related Deaths Kill More Than AIDS, TB, or Violence.[11]
- ✓ The cost of excessive alcohol use in the US rose to almost a quarter trillion dollars in 2010. The researchers believe that the study still underestimates the cost of excessive drinking because information on alcohol is often underreported or unavailable, and the study did not include other costs, such as pain and suffering due to alcohol-related injuries and diseases.[12]
- ✓ The 25.9% of underage drinkers who are alcohol abusers and alcohol dependent drink 47.3% of the alcohol that is consumed by all underage drinkers.[13] By the age of 16, most kids will have seen 75,000 ads for alcohol. Young people view 20,000 commercials each year, and nearly 2,000 of these are for beer and wine.[14]
- ✓ Alcohol is the most common drug among youth and a major contributor to morbidity and mortality worldwide. Billions of dollars are spent annually marketing alcohol.[15]

This is the product that so many Christian preachers and scholars either promote or refuse to condemn, and this is what (according to so many modern writers) Jesus, the LORD of the universe, created and drank at Cana!

On the other hand, there are an increasing number of Christian ministers and writers who do not promote this product and condemn moderate drinking for Christians without reserve. A recent posting on the internet, "Bible Wine," by Alathei Baptist Ministries is to be commended. They admit to the difficulty of promoting total abstinence, but they do so anyway:

> It would be an uphill battle merely to advocate moderation in drinking as many conservatives do, but to arrive at a conclusion that total abstinence is a biblical mandate, would place one immediately in the backwater of Christian social fellowships... [16]

In this book we will strongly advocate total abstinence, urging scriptural reasons as well as reasons that stem from the damage that alcohol is doing around the world and particularly in our country.

I. GRAPE JUICE IN THE BIBLE: CONTROVERSY!

It is a tragedy that, at a time when alcohol is causing more and more disasters in American society, there are is such wide and deep disagreement about what God has to say on the subject. In this book we will present the thesis that God clearly blesses grape juice in the Bible. We will also consider the subject of alcohol consumption in the Bible at length, for it seems inconceivable that the holy, righteous God would not teach His children clearly about such a dangerous subject. We must start by identifying the different teachings on the biblical meaning of wine and grape juice. The great many inconsistencies that are being taught today will be pointed out as will contradictions in the *teaching* of modern Bible scholars on this subject. Here are some of the differences that will be examined:

Many Bible teachers say that there is no fresh grape juice in the Bible:	Other reputable Bible scholars affirm the contrary:
The English Bible never mentions grape juice, the word "wine" in the Bible only refers to an alcoholic beverage.	The Bible speaks often of both grape juice and fermented wine, blessing the juice and clearly condemning the alcohol. The word for "wine" is often generic, meaning the fruit of the vine, and can be fresh grape juice or intoxicating wine.

The Bible permits moderate drinking of alcoholic beverages for God's people.	The Bible condemns drinking of alcoholic beverages for God's people and in no way condones it.
There was no safe drinking water in Palestine, and people had to mix an alcoholic beverage with water to make it safe.	There is no biblical, archaeological, or scientific evidence for this. The Bible reveals God's instructions for good sanitation and abounds with references to drinking water.
The Bible says that Jesus created and drank "wine," an alcoholic beverage.	Jesus could not have created or drunk a product that causes harm.

Who are the "some" that say there is no fresh grape juice in the Bible?

In Chapter VII, we will study more in depth the historical progression that has brought Christians in America to this controversy in the understanding of "grape juice" in the Bible. But here we have just summarized the differences between the "grapes" and "no grapes" or two-wines or one-wine understanding of the Bible, and now we will summarize just how we got to these diverse understandings.

Howard Crosby was one of the most followed early supporters of "no grape juice," or the "one-wine" position, as it is popularly called today. He was pastor of Fourth Avenue Presbyterian Church, New York City, and Chancellor of New York University beginning in 1870.

There are many articles, in "Christianity Today" and at least one in "The Baptist Bulletin," which carried information on "no grape juice," and soon it was taught even in fundamentalist Bible schools.

In 2008, Randy Jaeggli wrote and published *The Christian and Drinking, a Biblical Perspective on Moderation and Abstinence.* Interestingly, the book promoted the position of Abstinence for the Christian, while at the same time using all the arguments against the possibility of grape juice in the Bible. It was a popular book, used to promote moderate drinking, until its publishers took it out of circulation. It has been republished, but still holds the same position.

At the present time almost all Bible schools, even those in "fundamentalist" circles teach the one-wine position. However, there have been many "other" Bible teachers and authors who have taught and are teaching just the opposite.

Who are "other Bible scholars" who affirm the contrary?

The contrary of "one-wine" is "two-wine" and all those who declare that the Bible speaks of grape juice believe that there are two separate products, fermented and unfermented, which are found in the Bible.

Charles Welch was the first to question in writing the use of alcohol in the Lord's Supper. He did so in 1869.[17]

Frederick Lees was one of the first to study and write about grape juice in the Bible. He produced the Temperance Bible Commentary in 1870, where he separated every single passage dealing with "wine" in the Bible into two separate categories, "condemnations of the fermented kind and commendations of the unfermented kind."

George Marshall is one of the most interesting proponents of "grape juice" in Bible times. He was a leading judge and jurist in

Canada who became a Christian after studying the Scriptures in 1824. At that time, he was a great consumer of alcoholic beverages, but in studying the Bible, he was convinced that alcohol was not in God's plan for Christians, and immediately quit consuming. In 1855 he wrote *Strong Drink Delusion with Its Criminal and Ruinous Results Exposed*, which begins with the thesis that the Bible has to be the final authority on whether Christians should drink intoxicating beverages. He then says, "I am prepared to take the position and shall fully maintain it, that there is no authority or sanction whatever, in any part of the sacred volume, for the habitual or ordinary use as a beverage of wine, of an intoxicating quality, or any other kind of intoxicating drink."[18] He then goes on to write a lengthy, well-documented chapter, "On the Wines of Scripture" in which he documents from ancient writings the fact that there is in Scripture both fresh grape juice and intoxicating wine.

William Patton published *The Laws of Fermentation and the Wines of the Ancients* in 1871, a complete study of "wine" in the Bible, which soon sold out and was not republished until 2004.

Robert Teachout wrote his doctoral thesis, "The Use of 'Wine' in the Old Testament" in 1980 for Dallas Theological seminary. He studied every use of the word in Scripture from the original languages, and his conclusion was the same as those we have mentioned. He published a book, based on his research, *Wine, the Biblical Imperative: Total Abstinence* in 1983. He told me recently that during the writing of his thesis, he would not read any other books on the subject or make any conclusion until his study of wine in Scripture was completed.

How can there be such a huge difference in understanding of the meaning of one biblical word? How can this be? Chapter VII will extensively chronicle the great shifts in attitude towards consumption of alcohol in just 150 years here in the United States, both in society as a whole and especially in the Christian community. It can be briefly said here that society moved from having a majority who were convinced of the evil of drinking and worked very hard at combating it to the present era where the evil of drinking has been accepted as normal in society and the youth lead the way in "pushing the envelope." The Christian community went from preaching and teaching against the use of alcoholic beverages to the present situation in which many evangelical leaders promote moderate consumption, where most evangelicals neither fight it nor teach against it, and where very few evangelical churches aggressively practice abstinence. Furthermore, the teaching that grape juice is in the Bible is attacked by all but a very few Bible scholars.

How can there be so many serious contradictions in God's inspired Word as those found in the debate on "wine" in the Bible? I would affirm and insist that there are *never* contradictions in God's Word nor can there be. There are only contradictions in our interpretation or understanding of it.

We must start with the assurance and conviction that each Scriptural thought or word is to be interpreted

> There are no contradictions in God's Word-nor can there be-it is inspired and inerrant!

or understood in such a way that it can only complete and harmonize with the rest of Scripture. To be true to Himself, God must consistently speak the same truth throughout His Revelation! Therefore, in the case of the word "wine" in the Bible, we must work to find out what this word meant to its writers and readers in Bible times. Then we must apply that truth in our own lives, for "whatsoever things were written aforetime were written for our learning, that we through patience and comfort of the scriptures might have hope" (Rom. 15:4). "Hope" here does not mean wishful thinking but "joyful and confident expectation." Jeremiah speaks of God as being the hope of Israel (Jer. 17:13). The Psalmist says, "Happy is he that hath the God of Jacob for his help, whose hope is in the LORD his God" (Ps. 146:5). Our hope is more than salvation. It includes all that God has promised us of His blessing and protection in our lives. Our "hope" is absolutely vain if God does not speak objective truth, if He does not mean what He says. This hope can only be realized by accepting all that the Bible says and putting it into practice.

The uncompromising and public sniping at the biblical truth concerning the "grape juice-wine issue" has exponentially increased in our time. The central issue, the necessity of understanding God's Word always to be consistent, has always been clearly upheld by faithful men of God in our country, even in reference to grape juice in the Bible. Some of the confusion mentioned above comes from the fact that the Bible seems to bless and condemn the same beverage. As early as 1883, Leon Field pointed out this fact. He stated that in one class of passages the Bible clearly condemns this beverage and in another it commends it "in the strongest and most unmistakable language."[19] He added that it is described as a blessing and a curse, it is allowed and interdicted, and it is a symbol of spiritual blessings and an emblem of divine wrath. Of course, this is all very confusing if the word "wine" in the Bible only means a fermented beverage. But the Bible is clearly speaking of two wines in all its references, one of which is unfermented grape juice and the other which is fermented wine.

Eliphalet Nott, president of Union College in the early 1800s went even further than Field. When he spoke of the inconsistencies that would be evident if God blessed and condemned the same substance, he stated:

> Can the same thing in the same state be good and bad, a symbol of wrath, a symbol of mercy, a thing to be sought after, a thing to be avoided? Certainly not! And is the Bible then inconsistent with itself? No it is not, and this seeming inconsistency will vanish.[20]

Let us continue our present study with the goal of under-standing what God has to say about grape juice and alcoholic beverages. In order to do this, I feel I must share some of my experiences that have helped me in my search for the answers to the problem and have contributed to my present conclusion.

II. A PERSONAL PROBLEM WITH ALCOHOL

My personal problem with alcohol did not consist of using it occasionally or of becoming a slave to it. Instead, as I got older, it was an increasing uneasiness concerning what was being taught in Bible schools on the subject and how that affected my ministry.

I grew up in a home where the use of alcohol was a non-issue. We firmly believed that alcohol had no place in a Christian's life. I stayed with a Christian farmer and his wife in Pennsylvania during my high school years when my parents (who were missionaries) went back to Africa. No one that I knew in the church would have thought that alcoholic beverages had any place at all in a Christian home. Every single Sunday dinner in our house was accompanied by a radio program from Pacific Garden Mission in Chicago called "Unshackled." Most of their programs at that time were stories of professional men with families who started out with light or moderate social drinking and then went on to finally become down-and-out bums on skid row where they found the Savior and gave up their alcohol. I had no desire whatsoever to try alcohol for myself. After high school, I went to a fundamentalist Baptist seminary and then went into the Marine Corps, where alcohol was a major problem. Throughout this time, I was convinced that God did not condone alcohol for the Christian, but I would have been unable to answer the question about a Christian's right to drink alcohol because I had accepted what was taught in Bible School, that in Bible times it was impossible to keep grape juice fresh and that because of this, *wine* in the Bible was fermented.

My wife was brought up in a dysfunctional home because of an alcoholic father. Without going into details, she was the only one of the family who graduated from high school and then college. She had found the Lord during grade school and He preserved her during a very bad situation. Naturally, she has a strong aversion to any alcoholic beverage.

We met while I was still in the military service, married, and started a family. After three more years in the Marine Corps, including a stint in Vietnam, I mustered out of military service. During all my time in the USMC, I was never in the least tempted to taste any alcoholic beverage, though it literally flowed around me. My worst experiences during that time were seeing young marines from good families start moderately with alcohol and then go quickly downhill toward destruction in alcohol abuse and other sinful practices.

I left the military in order to go back to seminary and finish the last year of a five-year Th.B. degree. During that year in 1964, the Lord called us to the mission field. After that, I finished three years of graduate study in order to set up a seminary in the Central African Republic where we felt God was leading us.

After I finished graduate school, we went on to the Central African Republic and worked there seven years. In those churches, consumption of alcohol among Christians was never a problem. To be a Christian was to reject one's former practices and to live free from slavery to alcohol. When people accepted the Lord, they left their former habits, which had included much consumption of alcoholic beverages. On Saturday evenings, from miles around, we could hear the drums and the dances going on in the villages. These people were stimulated and maintained by local alcoholic beverages leading to all sorts of sexual debauchery. Those who accepted the gospel did not consider mixing their former slavery to sin and their new freedom in Christ.

After seven years in Africa, we began our ministry in France. It was a completely different scene from Africa. We had spent a year in France before leaving for Africa to learn the French language, and thus we understood the part that wine has had in the French culture. We knew that unfortunately most French Christians, just like their fellow citizens, consider that a meal without wine is not civilized.

We also knew that several American misconceptions of why alcoholic beverages are consumed by French Christians were simply not true. We had been told that the French drink wine because "they cannot get water that is safe to drink," but in France, wherever alcoholic beverages are sold, bottled water is always available-and much cheaper. We were also told that French Christians always dilute their wine to safe levels. This is simply not true. Sometime after we had moved from France to Quebec, we went back to visit. We were invited to a Christian wedding recep-tion that was attended by many who had been part of our former youth group and where the bride and groom also had been in our youth group. We knew most of the participants and guests well and were terribly saddened to see the wine flow copiously. In America a breathalyzer test would have kept them all from driving home legally. We decided then and there to never again attend a reception where alcohol would be served.

I served in France for seven years as pastor of a church. One Biblical subject we did not touch while in France was "wine" in the Bible. We had been told, by a veteran missionary on our arrival, that one must never tell a French Christian that one did not drink wine because of "principles" or "biblical convictions." Some other reason needed to be advanced. According to this missionary. We should never question their culture or the importance of wine in their daily life. This was very important to them.

During our time in France and in that church, we never accepted a drink and never had wine in our youth activities (though this

11

would have been the norm if I had not been the pastor), but I respected the protocol and never taught why the subject of "wine" in the Bible was important. I have felt badly since I left there that I had not been faithful to God in this respect. I did later give a copy of my book in French on the subject to each of the young people with whom I had had a teaching relationship.

While we lived in France, a myth was exploded for me, and my thinking was radically changed concerning "wine" in the Bible. I had believed from my youth that it was wrong for a Christian to drink alcohol. My family, my church, and my friends had shared that position and I felt comfortable in my conviction that this was what the Bible taught. I went to a Bible school, Baptist Bible Seminary, in Johnson City, New York, that also believed that alcohol was wrong for a Christian.

But they also taught at this school, as they were beginning to teach in others, that there was no grape juice in the Bible, because, simply and irrefutably, there was no way to preserve grape juice fresh in a hot climate. I had accepted this so irrevocably that I had simply laid aside a book I had read after graduation, a book that gave a clear teaching concerning "wine" in the Bible, which expounded the same view that I now hold. Though this book was well written and soundly researched, it simply would not compute with what I had been taught. I had accepted the "fact" that wine in the Bible could not be anything but an alcoholic beverage, since one could *not* preserve fresh grape juice in Biblical times!

Then, without researching the subject, something happened that blew the "facts" I had accepted into fragments and greatly kindled my interest. I was still in France, and one day my neighbor, who was not a Christian but who knew me well, offered me a drink of grape juice, as we were chatting in his cellar. It was August and well before the harvest time for his grapes. I knew he had grapevines in his garden and that he always made his own grape juice. When he offered me the glass that he poured from a corked jug that had been sitting on the floor, I looked at him with surprise and with questions. He said, "I know you do not drink wine. This is grape juice from my garden."

I said (stupidly), as I knew when he harvested his grapes, "You kept it fresh from last fall?" He said, "Bien sur," which means, "of course."

I asked, "How did you keep it fresh?"

He said, "I bring it to a boil, put it in a jug, put a cork in it, and leave it in my unheated cellar."

I let him know that I was very surprised, for I had always been taught that fresh grape juice would turn to alcohol. Then, wanting to know specifically if grape juice could be conserved for an entire year, from harvest to harvest, I asked him if I could have a drink from the same jug of last year's juice after his new grape juice was made.

He promised to call me at that time and did. Wow! What a shock! That which I had been told, taught, and believed, simply was not true! Grape juice *could* be kept fresh all year long with very minimum effort! From this point in my life, I began to study the subject in earnest. It would take a few years, but my "problem" of not understanding what God has to say about grape juice would finally disappear.

Now I will resume the story of my "re-education." I did not have the possibility of teaching on this matter during the rest of my stay in France.

After seven years in France, we went to Quebec, Canada, where I taught in a Baptist theological school and pastored Baptist churches for twenty years. During our early years there we saw a great shift in practice in the churches concerning alcohol. Wine is not the usual alcoholic beverage in Quebec, though alcoholic consumption (beer) has long been a real problem in their society. When the gospel first entered Quebec in 1948 and churches were started, it was generally taught that when a person was "saved," he was also to be delivered from alcohol. That was what was practiced and taught in the new churches that were established.

Unfortunately, within a few decades this situation changed, and the consumption of alcohol was being embraced by more and more Christians. In a very short period of time, an increasing number of Quebecker Christians were following English Christians in Canada and America toward allowing moderate alcoholic consumption. Only a small number of churches in Quebec continued to teach total abstinence. The change was rapid, and a response was needed. I wrote a book on the subject, *Le vin, la Bible, et le Chrétien*, which translates to English as *Wine, the Bible, and the Christian*. My goal was to offer Christians solid biblical proofs of God's consistent teaching on abstinence. These are the proofs I had not had in my earlier ministry but had so desperately needed. The book was not widely read, for alcohol is a big thing in Quebec society and Christians are relatively few. However, there was an effect. One young man in French Quebec wrote me 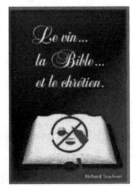 after my French book was published, "I was just about to start drinking alcohol moderately when I read your book, because I had read that the Bible said it was all right. Now I am a convinced non-drinker of alcohol."

During the writing of this book my education continued. Up until that time, all the books written about grape juice in the Bible were from America and American culture. I decided to search for a Canadian book on the subject. I went to the largest university in Quebec, University of Laval, not really expecting to find anything.

But I did! I found a book on microfilm that gave me a great step forward in understanding the problem. We have already mentioned the author, George Marshall, and the book that he wrote *Strong Drink Delusion, with Its Criminal and Ruinous Results*

Exposed. The amazing thing about this man was first, that it was the Word of God that convinced him alcohol was not for him in his new life as a Christian. Secondly. He was not satisfied with the teaching that there was no grape juice in the Bible, and he did an incredible amount of original research into written records from Bible times in several languages to prove his point. Finally, he travelled extensively to speak on the subject, at a time when travelling was difficult and expensive, to challenge great crowds in Canada, England and the USA.

During my entire ministry in these three foreign countries, my contact with America was infrequent, being limited to brief visits to my supporting churches. When I moved back to the US and began my ministry at Bibles International, I became aware of the tremendous change in the attitude of the Christian community toward alcohol. This change is detailed in Chapter XI. I also became aware of the aggressive teaching detailed in the Introduction which affirmed: "***The Bible never mentions grape juice; the word "wine" only refers to an alcoholic beverage.***" I found good churches that had church constitutions that included statements about abstinence for their members, but the practice was much different. Actual practice was, "the less said about this-the better." Finally, I found that the number of Christians who drank alcohol and who defended their right to do so was increasing dramatically and that those who believed that the Scriptures clearly taught abstinence did not have the resources to defend their position. This reality convinced me to pursue the study which has resulted in this book.

III. A KEY PROBLEM OF INTERPRETATION

The first question that we must resolve, in our search to resolve the controversy that was detailed in chapter I is, "what does the word "wine" mean in the Bible?" That which complicates the matter is the fact that most Christians would say, "We know what the word means-wine is wine-why should we even look further"? The answer is simple and complex, simple, because it will greatly influence our understanding of the proper attitude about alcohol, and complex because we have to go back in history to see what the English word has meant in the past and also examine the meaning of the. Hebrew and Greek words that were translated by "wine."

The popular and universal understanding of the English word *wine* in the Bible at the present time is that it is always understood to be an alcoholic beverage. Christians usually see no need for "interpreting" the Bible. Normally we just accept the general idea that "if it makes sense to me, then that is what it says." The trouble with that is that the Bible is God's spoken word, but spoken originally in Hebrew and Greek, in a different language from English, and to people that live in a different culture from our own. What we need to understand is what God's words meant to those that received them.

The understanding that wine is always alcoholic is not a proper understanding of the meaning of this word in Scripture. "Wine" is an English word, with a generic meaning, "the fruit of the vine," as we shall see. The Hebrew and Greek words translated by *wine* in our English Bibles often mean "fresh grape juice." How can this be? How can there be such a tremendous difference in the understanding of one word in the English Bible?

The specific problem of understanding what God says about grape juice and wine in the Bible is this: the English translation for seven Hebrew words and one Greek word is just one word, "wine," though there is a clear difference in meaning between the Hebrew words. In modern English, the word "wine" always means an alcoholic beverage. Our understanding of "wine" is, therefore, colored by our present American culture.

And yet, the answer to this specific problem of interpretation is quite simple-the English word "wine" in the English Bible as it was translated in the 17th century was different from our understanding today. It was a generic word then, meaning something which is general, common, or inclusive, rather than specific, unique, or selective. It meant very simply, "the fruit of the vine." Webster's 1828 Dictionary gave this primary meaning: "The expressed juice of grapes." This means that it is one word which can mean at least two kinds of drinks, both grape juice and fermented wine.

This is certainly not the only case in the English language where a word has two different meanings. The word "water" is an example of this, for we have to specify saltwater, fresh water, hard water, and unsafe drinking water, to express fully our meaning.

Another very good example of a generic word is the English word "cider." Cider is the juice pressed from fruits (apples, for example) which can be used for drinking or making other products such as vinegar. When I was a teenager on a farm in Pennsylvania, we made it and drank it every year, and it had *no* alcoholic content. Yet for many, apple cider is "hard cider" made from apple juice but fermented. Webster's on-line dictionary says, "Cider is an unfiltered juice or fermented beverage made from apples. In the fall, there's nothing like a mug of hot, spiced cider." We know the definition, but always in Quebec and even in some restaurants in the USA, when you ask for cider, you will get hard cider.

The English word "wine" in the Bible is just such a generic word meaning the fruit of the vine in either form, grape juice or fermented wine. We will first have to decide if this is true. We will prove that here by looking at four different arguments.

1. That there is grape juice in the Bible is evident from Scriptural context.

The truth that the English word "wine" has more than one meaning is seen from the fact that although there are cases where "wine" must mean an alcoholic beverage in the Bible, because of the clear context in which it is used, there are also a great number of instances throughout Scripture where "wine" is clearly to be understood by unfermented grape juice.

Here are a few of these: (1) "wine" is spoken of as the fruit of the land (Deuteronomy 7:13), which is grape juice. Fermented wine is man-made, by a process; it is not a natural process, (2) "wine" in the Bible is often said to be furnished "out of the winepress"[21] (Deuteronomy 15:14), but that which is pressed out of grapes in the press is, of course, grape juice, and (3) the word "wine-press" is found fourteen times in the Bible and obviously 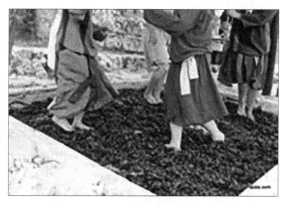 means "grape press," for they would put fresh grapes in a large container and crush them with their bare feet (as we have seen done in France).

It was considered to be a divine blessing, since they would gather in the grapes and produce its juice and with their corn and their oil. They felt successful, as corn and oil are mentioned often with wine as staples in their diet (Deuteronomy 11:14). As

Proverbs 3:10 mentions this blessing: "their presses would burst out with it." Conversely, God's judgment on Israel, spoken of in Isaiah 16:10, was severe: "the treaders shall tread out no wine in their presses." "Wine" here is grape juice, because it is obvious, that if you put fresh grapes in a container and press the juice out with your feet, it is fresh grape juice that comes out! Another very clear reference to fresh grape juice is Isaiah 65:8 where God says: "Thus saith the LORD, as the new wine is found in the cluster, and one saith, destroy it not; for a blessing is in it..." This means the fresh juice that is in the bunches of grapes.

2. That there is grape juice in the Bible is evident from other languages which translate Hebrew words for "wine" as grape juice.

While it may not seem perfectly clear in our English Bibles, often other languages have made the obvious distinction between grape juice and alcohol. In Isaiah 65:8, the English Bible says, "As the new wine is found in the cluster," but the French Bible (Louis Segond) says: "*Quand il se trouve du jus dans une grappe...*", which means in English, "When juice is found in a bunch of grapes... "The French translation here is better than the English, for that is what the Hebrew word says and there is obviously no fermented wine in a cluster or bunch of grapes!

The Hebrew word *yayin,* used most often in the Old Testament for the fruit of the vine, is generic and is always rendered "wine" in our English Bibles. The two principal words after *yayin* are *tirosh* (38 times) and *asis* (5 times), which are also translated to English by "wine." The French Bible translates *tirosh* by *moût* (must) most of the time, and *asis* as such every time. The principal meaning of *moût* and *assis* is not generic but refers specifically to "must" or fresh grape juice. Since we are using the English word "must," which is a little-known word in present-day English, we will define it:

> Must (from the Latin vinum mustum, "young wine") is freshly pressed fruit juice (usually grape juice) that contains the skins, seeds, and stems of the fruit... Making must is the first step in wine-making. Because of its high glucose content, typically between 10 and 15%, must is also used as a sweetener in a variety of cuisines.[22]

It is clear that the word *moût* in French and "*must*" in English can only mean unfermented grape juice. The foremost French dictionary, Larousse, defines *moût* as "unfermented grape juice which constitutes the raw material for winemaking." Here are some of the places in the Bible where *tirosh* is used:

> All the best of the oil, and all the best of the wine (*tirosh*, lit. unfermented grape juice), and of the wheat, the first-fruits of them which they shall offer unto the LORD, them have I given thee, (Num. 18:12).

> And this your heave offering shall be reckoned unto you, as though it were the corn of the threshing floor, and as the fulness (*tirosh*, lit. unfermented grape juice) of the winepress, (Num. 18:27).

> And he will love thee, and bless thee, and multiply thee: he will also bless the fruit of thy womb, and the fruit of thy land, thy corn, and thy wine (*tirosh*, lit. unfermented grape juice), and thine oil, the

> increase of thy kine, and the flocks of thy sheep,...
> (Deut. 7:13).

> Israel then shall dwell in safety alone: the foun-
> tain of Jacob shall be upon a land of corn and
> wine (*tirosh*, lit. unfermented grape juice); also his
> heavens shall drop down dew, (Deut. 33:28).

It is simply unscholarly to assert, as many modern writers do, that grape juice did not exist in ancient times and that it is not mentioned in the Bible. It is also not well to ignore the historical meaning of words, because words change in their meaning as time passes.

3. That there is grape juice in the Bible is evident from historical dictionary definitions.

The problem in understanding the original meaning of the biblical word *wine* is often caused by the fact that the English usage of the word *wine* has changed from that which was current in the 17th century in English, French, and Latin. Samuel Bacchiocchi says, after citing several sources:

> The above sampling of definitions of "wine" from
> older English dictionaries suggests that when the
> King James Version of the Bible was produced
> (1604-1611) its translators must have understood
> "wine" to refer to both fermented and unfer-
> mented wine.[23]

Actually, there are several books that show the undeniable fact that the Hebrew and Greek words for "wine" and their English and French translations have, down through history, been generic words referring to the fruit of the vine and what is done with it. Baker says, "On this point there can be little argument; it is certain that people in the ancient world drank grape juice, and oinos was sometimes used to refer to fresh, non-alcoholic wine."[24] Robert Teachout says,

> Long before the controversy over the prohibition against wine began in England and America, a large Latin lexicon, Thesaurus Linguae Latinae, (1740 AD) entered the fray. Volume 4, p. 557, gave several definitions for vinum [wine], all supported by ancient Roman texts, including "fresh grape juice," "bottled grape juice" and "grape juice (vinum)" so called while it was still in the unpressed grape.[25]

This generic use of the word wine and the French word "vin" can also be shown from older English, Italian and French dictionaries. Webster's Revised Unabridged Dictionary (1828 and 1913) gave this primary meaning: 1. the expressed juice of grapes, especially when fermented; a beverage or liquor prepared from grapes by squeezing out their juice, and (usually) allowing it to ferment.[26] If the fact that the words for wine in the Bible are generic is accepted, then it is easy to understand in any biblical context exactly what God is saying. If He blesses its production or use, He is talking about unfermented grape juice. If He condemns or curses its use, He is referring to the alcoholic beverage.

4. That there is grape juice in the Bible is evident from Bible stories.

One of the most striking examples of "wine" in the Bible being non-fermented concentrated grape juice is found in 1Samuel 25:18:

> Then Abigail made haste, and took two hundred loaves, and two bottles of wine, and five sheep ready dressed, and five measures of parched corn, and an hundred clusters of raisins, and two hundred cakes of figs, and laid them on asses.

She took all of that to provide for David's men, all 600 of them. Each item in the list was sufficient for the number of men in David's camp-except the two bottles of wine. If it was alcoholic wine, two bottles would 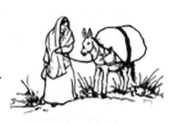 never suffice for so many men. No, it could only be two skins of concentrated grape syrup, which when mixed with water, would have provided sufficient sweet juice for all those men.

The story of Abigail's treat for David and his men is not the only biblical story, which shows the use of highly concentrated grape juice. 2 Samuel 16:1 tells the story of Ziba the servant of Mephibosheth, who met David on his return from a brief exile from Jerusalem. Ziba went out with a couple of asses, bearing two hundred loaves of bread, an hundred bunches of raisins, an hundred bunches of summer fruits, and a bottle of wine. That could not be one bottle or skin of alcoholic wine for all of David's men. It had to be concentrated grape juice that, when mixed with water, produced a soothing and delicious drink. Concentrated grape juice is abundantly used in many countries, even to the present time, and to my personal knowledge, specifically in France and Italy. The bottle pictured at the right and described below was listed at $19.00 a bottle!

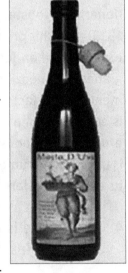

This unique grape beverage has been produced for centuries in the Italian region of Emilia Romagna. The ancient craft of slowly cooking fresh grape juice (in Italian, Mosto d'Uva) in huge kettles and reducing it to a rich liquid is being preserved by artisans like Adriano Guerzoni and his sons."[27]

My wife and I were familiar with concentrated grape juice when we lived in Africa and France. We were often served this highly concentrated juice, called *syrop* in French, which would be syrup in English. The first time we tasted of this was when we were invited into a French home in Africa. There we were served a delicious drink, where a quarter of an inch of concentrated grape syrup was poured into a glass, which was then filled with water. When we moved to France, a few years later, we found that this "syrop" (highly concentrated grape juice) was a regular part of French culture.

From these four arguments we can conclude from Scripture that grape juice is often mentioned in Scripture. It cannot therefore be true that "wine" in the Bible always means an alcoholic drink. It is rather true that when the English translation says "wine," it is generic in that "wine" refers to either grape juice or an alcoholic beverage. Grape juice is clearly present in the Scriptural account of Israel's daily life in the Promised Land. It cannot, therefore, be true that grape juice was never mentioned in the Bible. In our next chapter, we will look at Scripture and we will see how God blesses grape juice.

IV. GOD BLESSES THE NATURAL FRUIT OF THE VINE

L et us look at what God taught His people. Even before He brought them into the Promised Land, He gave them instructions that would enable them to lead a happy and prosperous life in that land. We find very specific instructions in Exodus through Deuteronomy. Just before the people entered Canaan, Moses gave a charge in Deuteronomy 27 and 28. He specifically detailed the effect that obedience or disobedience to His commandments would have on their lives.

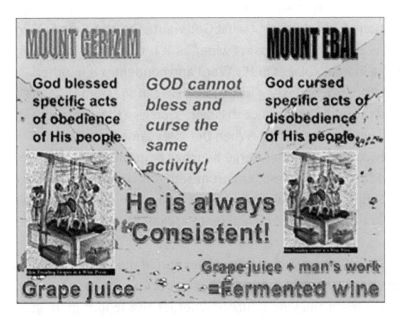

He does not in this passage mention *all* the activities that His children could do that would please Him and be blessed or would displease him and be cursed.

He does not specifically mention drinking "wine" here in the activities that he condemned. He simply says that if they are not obedient to all of His commandments, their vines would not produce: "Thou shalt plant vineyards, and dress them, but shalt neither drink of the wine, nor gather the grapes; for the worms shall eat them"(Deut. 28:39). "Wine" here is the Hebrew word *yayin* which is generic.

According to what we have shown in Chapter I, the most likely translation here is "grape juice." God is saying that if Israel does not obey His commandments, the grapevines and the grape juice with which He had promised to bless them would be taken away.

Why is it important to understand the use of the word "wine" in the Bible? God never, in all Scripture, contradicts Himself in blessing and in condemning the same thing. We will look at many biblical passages which seems to do just that. The following illustration would affirm that what God wanted to bless was only grape juice. He certainly blesses "wine," as it is translated in the English Bible in many places in His Word and condemns it in others.

As to God's blessing grape juice, we can see from Scripture that God promised grape juice to Israel: "God give thee... plenty of corn and wine" (Gen. 27:28). When the spies came back from their visit, they carried extremely large bunches of grapes as proof that this was the land that God had promised. It is clear from this portion of Scripture and many others that God planned for His people to have this healthy beverage (grape juice) for He mentions it 124 times in the Old Testament![28]

"Vine" and "vineyards" are mentioned nine times in just eight chapters in Song of Solomon! "Let us get up early to the vineyards; let us see if the vine flourish, whether the tender grape appear, and the pomegranates bud forth: there will I give thee my loves" (Song of Solomon 7:12). Vineyards and grapes were blessed by God and important to the Jews. In each vineyard there was provision for a wine press for the production of grape juice. In Scripture we find four actions of God in relation to His people which prove His blessing upon this natural product.

On the other hand, drinking "fermented wine" was condemned by God. In the next chapter we will discuss this in detail. Here we will simply cite three passages of Scripture that demonstrate this:

> Wine is a mocker, strong drink is raging; and whosoever is deceived thereby is not wise (Prov. 20:1).

> Who hath woe? who hath sorrow? who hath contentions? who hath babbling? who hath wounds without cause? who hath redness of eyes? They that tarry long at the wine... (Prov. 23:29, 30).

> They grope in the dark without light, and he maketh them to stagger like a drunken man (Job 12:25).

Those who cannot accept that God speaks of grape juice in the Bible do not understand a large part of the everyday life of His people in Bible times. God talks of both grape juice and alcoholic beverages: He blesses the first and condemns the use of the second. Below, we will give four acts of God in Scripture that demonstrate His intentional blessing of His people with the provision of grape juice.

1. God promised His people He would provide grape juice.

The Bible talks of "wine" as being God's blessed provision, a staple of the diet of His people even before they arrived in the Promised Land. Isaac promised Jacob: "Therefore God give thee of the dew of heaven, and the fatness of the earth, and plenty of corn and wine" (Gen. 27:28). God repeated this promise through the words of Joseph:

The sceptre shall not depart from Judah, nor a lawgiver from between his feet, until Shiloh come; and unto him shall the gathering of the people be. Binding his foal unto the vine, and his ass's colt unto the choice vine; he washed his garments in wine, and his clothes in the blood of grapes" (Gen. 49:10, 11).

God promised again through Moses:

"And he will love thee, and bless thee, and multiply thee: he will also bless the fruit of thy womb, and the fruit of thy land, thy corn, and thy wine, and thine oil, the increase of thy kine, and the flocks of thy sheep, in the land which he sware unto thy fathers to give thee" (Deut. 7:13).

The Israelites did not always appreciate God's blessing. One of many other examples of this in Scripture is the rebellion of Israel when they were about to enter the Promised Land. God had promised them this land (a great blessing), He had showed His mighty power in taking them out of Egypt, He had provided their needs (food and water), He had allowed the spies to go and check out this Promised Land. And His people whimpered: "there are giants in the land. We are going back to Egypt!"

Later in their history God said to the prophet Hosea concerning Israel that He had given them wine: "For she did not know that I gave her corn, and wine, and oil,..." (Hos. 2:8). He says in Psalm 104:13-15:

He watereth the hills from his chambers: the earth is satisfied with the fruit of thy works. He causeth the grass to grow for the cattle, and herb for the

service of man: that he may bring forth food out of
the earth; And wine that maketh glad the heart of
man, and oil to make his face to shine, and bread
which strengtheneth man's heart.

It can be seen from all of these citations that grape juice was
a basic and very important part of the diet in biblical times, as it is
very often mentioned with corn and oil or with bread.

Perhaps even more important to our study is the fact that
God's promises were made to Israel in the distant past, at the com-
mencement of their sojourn in the Promised Land. This became
an important part of their culture. When I drove northward out of
Jerusalem, in Palestine in my visit there, the mountainsides were
covered with what used to be terraced vineyards.

2. God predicted His provision of grape juice for His people long before their entry into the Promised Land

Did you ever wonder why the spies who brought back such a
glowing report of the Promised Land also brought back bunches
of grapes? Because, as we
have seen, God had promised
this blessing to Israel long
before they reached the point
of entering Canaan. We find
this promise detailed in
Deuteronomy 11:14, "That I
will give you the rain of your
land in his due season, the first rain and the latter rain, that thou
mayest gather in thy corn, and thy wine, and thine oil."

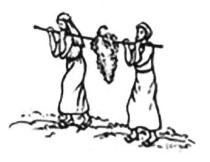

Now, as they were set to enter the Promised Land, God wanted
to encourage His people-even before they arrived in their new
home-with the proof that the land was producing exactly what He

had promised. Unfortunately, they rebelled and would not enter the land. They could only think of the enemies (the giants) they would have to face, and the grapes would have to wait.

3. God provided grape juice for the health and joy of His people.

Grapes and grape juice were very important to people in Bible times and were easily accessible. This we know because the Bible talks much of vines and vineyards. The fresh juice was a wonderful treat.

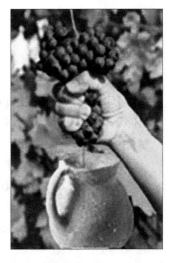

One of the earliest references to grape juice is found in Genesis 40:11: "And Pharaoh's cup was in my hand: and I took the grapes, and pressed them into Pharaoh's cup, and I gave the cup into Pharaoh's hand." Though the word used here in Scripture is still "wine," this is still very much grape juice, for it was the juice squeezed out of grapes.

Josephus, a Jewish historian from the time of Christ in his *Antiquities of the Jews*, chapter five, says: "he squeezed them into a cup which the king held in his hand; and when he had strained the wine, he gave it to the king to drink."[29] The Adam Clark Commentary in 1810 said this:

> From this we find that wine anciently was the mere expressed juice of the grape, without fermentation. The saky, or cup-bearer, took the bunch, pressed the juice into the cup, and instantly delivered it into the hands of his master. This was anciently the

32

yayin of the Hebrews, the oinos, of the Greeks, and
the mustum of the ancient Latins.[30]

The Bible talks often of this treat of freshly squeezed grape
juice as illustrated by Isaiah 65:8: "Thus saith the LORD, As the new
wine is found in the cluster,… a blessing is in it." Albert Barnes, a
noted Preacher and Bible Scholar, whose books are still very popular, says, "The Hebrew word (tirosh) used here means properly
must, or new wine."[31]

In one list of great blessings promised, God says: "Butter of
kine, and milk of sheep, with fat of lambs, and rams of the breed
of Bashan, and goats, with the fat of kidneys of wheat; and thou
didst drink the pure blood of the grape" (Deut. 32:14). At that
time, they did not have many sources of sugar, an important ele-
ment in diet. They had no candy, jam, ice cream, soft drinks, or
juice drinks! Grape juice in all its forms, concentrated or full, provided a large part of their need for sugar, as well as providing a
treat. We will see later on in our study of the process of making
alcoholic wine that sugar was not present in fermented wine as
the process of fermentation eliminates sugar. If, as many teach,
"wine" in Bible times was always fermented, then there would be
no fresh grape juice and they would not have the sugar needed
in the diet! Thus, grapes and their juice provide sugar and were
a very important part of meals as well as special treats for family
activities and voyages.

4. He proclaimed the use of it for the fellowship of His people.

In the Old Testament God constantly encourages the importance and wellbeing of the family. A strong, healthy family was the result of the practice of the Jewish faith. One of the important parts of that practice was the system of feasts established by God where the families were to unite regularly at home, at the tabernacle, or at the temple to fellowship with God and with each other. In these feast times, "wine" is said to have played a large part. God gave instructions for those who lived close to the temple and for those who lived far away, both of whom were required to present themselves before the Lord. For those who lived nearby:

> And thou shalt eat before the LORD thy God, in the place which he shall choose to place his name there, the tithe of thy corn, of thy wine, and of thine oil, and the firstlings of thy herds and of thy flocks; that thou mayest learn to fear the LORD thy God always (Deut. 14:23).

For those who lived far away, they were to sell their produce in their homes and bring the money to the temple:

> And thou shalt bestow that money for whatsoever thy soul lusteth after, for oxen, or for sheep, or for wine, or for strong drink, or for whatsoever thy soul desireth: and thou shalt eat there before the LORD thy God, and thou shalt rejoice, thou, and thine household, (Deut. 14:26).

If this "wine" was not grape juice, there is a problem of consistency in the instructions for sacrifices and feasts. Not only are there instances in Scripture where priests are commanded to both drink and not drink "wine," but Israel was told to bring both "wine" and "strong drink" as an offering to the Lord. Numbers 15:7 says: "And for a drink offering thou shalt offer the third part of an hin of wine, for a sweet savour unto the LORD." These passages make perfect sense if we understand them to be talking about grape juice. The Bible goes on to speak many times of "wine" (not fermented) used as an offering. Scripture also makes it very clear that leaven was not to be used in offerings and it is always present in fermented wine. Leaven, or yeast, is a substance used to cause fermentation. Grape juice has no leaven. Therefore, we can easily understand that He would permit only non-fermented grape juice for His drink offerings.

God can only bless natural grape juice, not alcoholic wine. In His Word He reveals the importance of this healthy drink by promising it to His people and by providing it for their enjoyment during times of worship and socializing.

V. PRESERVING GRAPE JUICE, IN BIBLE TIMES

We have seen from many Scriptures that grape juice was indeed spoken of in the Bible, but this immediately raises the question, "How did they keep it unspoiled and fresh?" This requires more information.

John George Marshall wrote in 1855 a book about "wine" in the Bible, in which he detailed proof for the preservation of grape juice:

> Several modes were known in the vine countries of the East, and were very generally practiced, for preserving the "fruit," or liquid of the grape from fermentation; and keeping it in that state, sweet, and free from the intoxicating quality, for any time desired. The chief mode it appears, [was],-boiling down the juice of the grape to syrup ...[32]

Actually, there are at least four methods of preserving grape juice fresh.

1. Boiling.

By evaporating most of the water, the consistency is made into a syrup, and the sugar content is too high a ratio. For this reason, it will not ferment. Tom Brennan cites three authors:[33]

> Herman Boerhave, Elements of Chemistry, 1668: By boiling, the juice of the richest grapes loses all its aptitude for fermentation, and may afterwards

Two Wines: A Proper Understanding of "Wine" in the Bible

be preserved for years without undergoing any further change.

Parkinson, Theatrum Batanicum, 1640: The juice or liquor pressed out of the ripe grapes is called vinum (wine). Of it is made both sapa and defrutum, in English cute, that is to say boiled wine, the latter boiled down to the half, or former to the third part.

William Patton, *Bible Wines,* 1874: Archbishop Potter, born AD 1674, in his *Greek Antiquities,* Edinburgh edition, 1813 says, vol. ii. p. 360, "The Lacedaemonians used to boil their wines upon the fire till the fifth part was consumed."

2. Filtration.

When the yeast, or leaven is filtered from the grape juice, one may prevent fermentation. The historian Plutarch writes (cited by Patton):

Wine is rendered old and feeble in strength when frequently filtered. The strength or spirit being thus excluded, the wine neither inflames the brain neither infests the mind and the passions and is much more pleasant to drink.[34]

3. Subsidence.

When permitting the leaven to settle, then pouring off the juice remaining, the gluten (another word for leaven or yeast) can be removed. Patton says,

Chemical science teaches that the gluten may be so effectually separated from the juice by subsidence as to prevent fermentation... He then quotes Calumello, "Gather the grapes and expose them for three days to the sun; on the fourth, at mid-day, tread them; take the museum lixivium; that is, the juice which flows into the lake before you use the press, and, when it has settled, add one ounce of powdered iris; strain the wine from its faces, and pour it into a vessel."[35]

4. Fumigation.

Fermentation can be prevented by introducing small amounts of Sulphur into the juice, or into the container. One simple way of doing this is to add a small amount of chicken eggs to the mixture.

Adams in his Roman Antiquities, on the authority of Pliny and others, says " that the Romans fumigated their wines with the fumes of sulphur; that they also mixed with the mustum, newly pressed juice, yolks of eggs, and other articles containing sulphur.[36]

It is then obvious that the ancient world knew several ways to preserve grape juice fresh and considered it so important that their many writings have come down to us.

Marshall also cites a celebrated oriental traveler that he met in Edinburgh who "stated that the Mahometans (Muslims) to whom intoxicating drink of any kind is forbidden, carried with them in their journeys the unfermented wine."[37] We can add that the Koran clearly outlaws alcoholic wine for all Muslims and yet blesses grapes and their production, which obviously shows that they could preserve it. Here is an interesting quote from a Muslim source on the internet, *Islam, Question & Answer*:[38]

> Drinking alcohol is a major sin, for wine is the
> mother of all evils. It clouds the mind, wastes
> money, causes headaches, tastes foul, and is an
> abomination of the Shaytaan's [Satan's] handiwork.
> It creates enmity and hatred between people, pre-
> vents them from remembering Allaah and praying,
> calls them to zina [unlawful sexual relationships],
> and may even call them to commit incest with their
> daughters, sisters or other female relatives.

In the first chapter, I told of experiencing first-hand the way to preserve grape juice, which goes back to Bible times. In fact, there are many modern authors who document a great many ancient methods of preservation. The easiest was to keep the juice fresh by simply bringing it to a boil and then sealing it in a bottle or jug and keeping it in a cellar or cave. Also, they could boil the syrup down to a paste which was easy to carry. Of course, they could also preserve the grapes whole in order to make their juice later in the year.[39]

Jennifer Woodruff wrote an interesting article in *Christianity Today*, "Raise a Juice Box to the Temperance Movement," in which she speaks of the beginning of the availability of grape juice in the American market (Welches Grape Juice). She stated that Louis Pasteur had proved that heating grape juice to a temperature of 140 to 212 degrees Fahrenheit killed bacteria and molds and yeast. Pasteur used this process to inject exactly the yeast he wanted for the wine he wanted. She says;

> But T. B. and Charles [Welch] wanted to halt the
> process right after the pasteurizing: no yeast, no
> fermentation. They picked grapes from the trellis
> outside their house, cooked them, filtered them,
> and plunged the bottles of cooked and filtered juice

into boiling water-keeping them in there not too long, but just long enough.

When the bottles were uncorked, they had not fermented. T. B. had succeeded.[40]

It is quite obvious that the ancients had the same means of keeping grape juice fresh as did Welch.

Field discusses other, more technical, means of preserving grape juice in Bible times, always citing Roman and Greek writers from that epoch.[41]

It is interesting that Field and many from his time and from the present time present their work in a very scholarly fashion, unlike those of their time and the present time who totally deny those findings.

Besides information from antiquity, there is much information on the internet on making grape juice and preserving it. One such is a post from Michigan State University in which their recipe is very simple. They say that one must pick the grapes, wash them, and put them in a pan with boiling water to heat, and then use a canning process.

At this point, we repeat that the number one proof advanced by all those who insist that "wine" in the Bible is *always* intoxicating. This "proof" is simple: they maintain that since there was no refrigeration in ancient times, there could be no preservation of natural grape juice. As we have seen, this is not true.

I had an interview and an extended conversation with Randy Jaeggli, author of the most popular book that promotes the "fact," of only fermented wine in the Bible. We conversed in a room in Bob Jones University. He had a friend with him, a PhD from the science department, and I had a friend with me, a pastor who was vitally interested in the subject. Dr. Jaeggli and his friend both clung to their "fact" or "proof" and would not accept any arguments against it that I could advance.

And yet, there are a great many books written, going back to Bible times, that refute their proof or fact that "wine" in the Bible is ALWAYS intoxicating.

VI. GOD'S PROBLEM WITH ALCOHOL

Throughout the Old Testament we read how God blesses "wine" which is grape juice in the Bible. However, in the Scriptures God reveals that He has a major problem with "wine" which is fermented. He very specifically talks about its effects on the human body. It is easy to see in Scripture that there is a world of difference between the natural juice of a natural fruit and man-made alcohol that is made by adding something to the juice which changes it completely.

In 1919 Richmond Pearson Hobson published a book, *Alcohol and the Human Race*. He, as a member of Congress, was urged by his political advisors to vote against a Prohibition amendment. He resisted the tremendous pressure that was building against the Prohibition movement and decided to study all that was available in the Library of Congress. This is what he said about his findings:

> I was startled to find, almost at the outset, that alcohol is not a product built up of grain, grapes and other food materials, but is the toxin of yeast or ferment germs, which, after devouring the food materials, excrete alcohol as their waste product[42]

We must never forget that in all discussion of wine in the Bible, if it is a fermented drink, it is NOT a natural drink. It is a man-made, poisonous, product. Let's examine two things Christians often say today about wine:

1. "If you wait just a little bit, grape juice turns to wine."
2. "Since God made wine, then it is good for us. Let us partake!"

Nothing could be further from the truth than to think that grape juice turns to wine automatically. If you put a glass of grape juice in the kitchen window, it will not turn to grape juice or vinegar, it will simply spoil and smell. This is something the reader can try for himself. I have.

God did not *make* wine. It is always a *process* that man uses to make fermented wine that was discovered centuries ago. There are many descriptions on the internet to describe how wine is made and even how to make wine at home. The start for any wine-making project, after selecting the grapes and crushing them, creating must (fresh grape juice with the skins), is to add yeast or leaven. This must be present.

The yeast converts the sugar into ethanol (alcohol) and carbon dioxide, which disappears. After the fermentation process, which can take different periods of time, according to the instructions, the alcoholic wine is stored in different ways.

Grape juice, which is not treated, either boiled to concentrate the sugar content or fermented to make alcohol, will simply spoil and smell. However, treating grape juice to preserve it as grape juice was and is relatively easy. Much is written in Roman and Greek writings about the use of preserved grape juice:

> **Defrutum**, **carenum**, and **sapa** were reductions of must used in Roman cuisine. They were made by boiling down grape juice or must (freshly squeezed grapes) in large kettles until it had been reduced to two-thirds the original volume, carenum; half the original volume, defrutum; and one-third, sapa. The main culinary use of defrutum was to help preserve and sweeten wine, but it was also added to fruit and meat dishes as a sweetening and souring agent and even given to food animals

such as suckling pig and duck to improve the taste of their flesh.[43]

This and other historical references to boiled "must" simply show that it was available in Bible times and was easily preserved as concentrated, non-alcoholic grape juice.

God did not make wine. He made grapes, from which comes grape juice. It was man that created wine. William Patton, the earliest writer on this subject in modern times, cites many authorities of his time concerning this. I will quote two of these:

> Sir Humphrey Davy says of alcohol: "It has never been found ready formed in plants." Count Chaptal, the eminent French chemist, says: "Nature never made spirituous liquors: she rots the grape upon the branch, but it is art which converts the juice into (alcoholic) wine."[44]

Instead of being a God-given, pure, natural juice, wine is a poisonous product made by man. We will discuss this later in more detail, but first consider two statements from the internet: One article says (October 2018): Alcohol causes more harm than many less legal substances.[45] Another article (August 2018) says: "Alcohol is a leading cause of death and disease worldwide."[46] This article declares that alcohol, such as beer and wine, is a leading risk factor for death and disease, associated with 2.8 million deaths each year and the seventh-leading risk factor for premature death and disability globally in 2016.

In light of the known effects of alcohol on the human body, it would be surprising if God did not have much to say about this-and He does!

Stephen M. Reynolds, PhD, graduate of Princeton University, a recognized authority on biblical languages wrote *The Biblical*

Approach to Alcohol in 2003. In his book, he treated a great many passages of Scripture with his extensive knowledge of the biblical languages to find out the truth in the one-wine-two-wine debate, and he shows throughout his book that the two-wine understanding is correct. He often refers to Proverbs 23:29-32 as being the definitive commandment in Scripture to not look at or consider or touch fermented wine.[47] He believes, by the Hebrew words used, that this passage is a commandment to all, that it is assuredly talking of fermented wine, and that it gives an excellent understanding of the danger of alcohol and the effects it has on the body. It is interesting to note that this condemnation of fermented wine is found in the immediate context of God's severe condemnation of adultery, a. sin that God clearly abhors and constantly speaks to in Scripture.

Here is God's commandment (Prov. 23:29-32):

> Who hath woe? who hath sorrow? who hath contentions?
>
> who hath babbling? who hath wounds without cause?
>
> who hath redness of eyes? They that tarry long at the wine;
>
> they that go to seek mixed wine.
>
> Look not thou upon the wine when it is red[48],
>
> when it giveth his colour in the cup,
>
> when it moveth itself aright.
>
> At the last it biteth like a serpent,
>
> and stingeth like an adder.

God continually condemns "wine" in Scripture:

> Wine is a mocker, strong drink is raging; and whosoever is deceived thereby is not wise (Prov. 20:1).

> They grope in the dark without light, and he maketh them to stagger like a drunken man (Job 12:25).

> Woe unto them that are mighty to drink wine… (Isa. 5:22)

> Woe unto them that rise up early in the morning, that they may follow strong drink; that continue until night, till wine inflame them! (Isa. 5:11).

> Let us walk honestly, as in the day; not in rioting and drunkenness… (Rom. 13:13).

> And be not drunk with wine, wherein is excess…. (Eph. 5:18).

God commands the priests not to drink wine:

> Do not drink wine nor strong drink, thou, nor thy sons with thee, when ye go into the tabernacle of the congregation, lest ye die: (Lev. 10:9).

God describes wine as poison:

> Their wine is the poison of dragons, and the cruel venom of asps (Deut. 32:33).

God talks of those who were "drunken" and what they did: Noah contributed to the sin of his son because he was under the influence of alcohol: "And he drank of the wine and was drunken …" (Gen. 9:21).

Lot drank and sinned:

> And they made their father drink wine that night:
> and the firstborn went in and lay with her father;
> and he perceived not when she lay down, nor when
> she arose (Gen. 19:33).

Eli was used to seeing people under the influence: "And Eli said unto her, how long wilt thou be drunken? put away thy wine from thee." (1 Sam. 1:14)

Nabal's drinking cost him his life: "Nabal's heart was merry within him, for he was very drunken…. And it came to pass about ten days after, that the Lord smote Nabal, that he died" (1 Sam. 25:36-38).

Amnon too, died when his heart was "merry with wine" (2 Sam. 13:28).

Ahasuerus tried to subject his queen, Vashti, to public humiliation in displaying her beauty before his guests. This was counter to usual practice; in their culture one did not parade one's wife before other men! He would never have done this while sober, but in this case, he had drunk too much alcohol:

> And they gave them drink in vessels of gold,… and
> royal wine in abundance…. On the seventh day,
> when the heart of the king was merry with wine,
> he commanded…. to bring Vashti the queen before
> the king with the crown royal, to shew the people
> and the princes her beauty: for she was fair to look
> on. (Esther 1:7, 10, 11).

In Proverbs 4:17, God characterizes wine as promoting violence: "For they eat the bread of wickedness and drink the wine of violence." We can certainly relate to this in our day. Almost every day our local television has at least one story of deaths and harm resulting directly from alcohol. This is such a usual thing that, after headlining an accident or incident of violence where alcohol was not the cause, the reporter will specify this.

In summarizing the teaching from all the passages in the Bible that speak of alcohol, we find that God severely condemns alcoholic beverages for His people for the following reasons:

- it keeps one who drinks from drawing near to God;
- it deceives one who drinks-we know now that the very first drink goes directly to the brain and reduces a person's resistance to sin;
- it inflames one who drinks;
- it causes one who drinks to err and to stumble;
- it causes one who drinks to stagger;
- it causes one who drinks to be poor;
- it causes one who drinks to sin;
- it causes one who drinks to be violent.

There are a great many stories on the internet about the effects of alcohol. They can be googled by choosing "stories about recovery from alcoholism." They show the effects of alcohol and the difficulty of recovering over and over and over. Most of these stories show that the beginning of the downfall was with alcohol at a very young age and then graduated to drugs. That which is *not* found on the internet is the terrible end of the story for all those who did not recover.

God's problem with alcoholic wine is that it is poison and when one drank it, his body is affected adversely. The solution seems pretty simple: don't drink it. When people speak to me and say, "... but wine in the Bible was highly diluted and was not nearly as alcoholic as now...". I simply answer, "But in the Bible, even with weaker wine, people got drunk when they drank it!" God warns where that leads. Some would say, why consider God's warning?

49

I would answer that in our present society we realize that all the warnings from family and society and all the scientific and specific statistics as to the danger of alcohol does NOT keep young people from drinking. That drinking is bad is admitted even by those who were and are opposed to prohibition. Garrett Peck wrote a stinging criticism of Prohibition in his book "The Prohibition Hangover" and yet he has a long section on what is bad about alcohol, in which he says, "Alcohol is the most widely used drug in American society-and by far the most dangerous. It is our nation's largest addiction."[49]

The strongest motivation that can make a young person choose to not partake of alcohol is his personal conviction that God wants him to live a successful and heathy life and desires him to not drink that which causes so much pain and disaster. He cannot choose this if he is not taught this in his church and by his parents!

VII. A HISTORICAL PROBLEM WITH ALCOHOL IN AMERICA: A QUICK LOOK AT THE BATTLE FOR TEMPERANCE

We cannot properly understand the present bias against finding "grape juice" in the Bible or the actual tidal wave of Christians beginning to drink alcohol, without looking back in history to a time when this interpretational and practical battle was fought on a massive scale. That whole era is often called "Prohibition." Actually, it should include not just the actual time when Prohibition became the law of the land but also the battle for temperance that took place before, that was led by those who preached from the Word of God.

Today, the popular claim from both sides of the issue is that the law that banned the sale and production of alcoholic beverages was a total failure, because of the violence it engendered and the fact that it did not stop a lot of people from finding alcohol to drink. Mark Thornton wrote an article, "Alcohol Prohibition Was a Failure," in which he follows the accepted analysis of today:

> National prohibition of alcohol (1920-33)-the "noble experiment"--was undertaken to reduce crime and corruption, solve social problems, reduce the tax burden created by prisons and poorhouses, and improve health and hygiene in America. The results of that experiment clearly indicate that it was a miserable failure on all counts.[50]

Garrett Peck in his "Prohibition Hangover" says,

> Fox News's Eric Burns writes in The Spirits of
> America (2004): "the Eighteenth Amendment to
> the Constitution of the United States [was] perhaps
> the worst idea ever proposed by a legislative body
> anywhere in the world for the ostensible goal of a
> better society.[51]

However, this is a very inaccurate and short-sighted view. Not
only did Prohibition have a beneficial effect on society as a whole
at that time, but the Christian Bible teaching which greatly helped
to produce it also had a positive effect on Christianity that would
last a hundred years. This will be shown in Chapter XI.

Concerning the state of American society before Prohibition,
a historian said, in a book written in 1920:

> At the opening of the century it really seemed
> as if the manhood of America was about to be
> drowned in strong drink. The cheapness of untaxed
> intoxicants-rum, whiskey, and apple-jack, made
> by anyone who chose to undertake the business
> and sold at every gathering of the people without
> reference to the age or sex of the purchaser-had
> made drunkenness almost universal. Samuel Brech,
> writing at the close of the eighteenth century, says
> that "it was impossible to secure a servant-white
> or black, bond or free-who could be depended on
> to keep sober for twenty-four hours. All classes
> and professions were affected. The judge was

overcome on the bench; the minister sometimes
staggered on his way to the pulpit… "[52]

Rev. Lyman Beecher, who was describing the ordination of a
minister at Plymouth, Connecticut, in 1810, said,

At this ordination the preparation for our creature
comforts besides food included a broad sideboard
covered with decanters and bottles…. The drinking
was apparently universal… they always took something to drink around, also before public services,
and always on their return.[53]

Not only was society going down the slippery slope of more
and more consumption of alcohol, but many Christians followed
right along. This being the state of the church and Christianity, it is
a great wonder that Prohibition happened at all and that it accom-
plished anything at all.

An adequate history of the battles for abstinence cannot be
undertaken here. In this survey, the epoch will be summarized
with cameos of some of the preachers of the time who worked
very hard to teach God's Word on the subject as well as some
preachers and writers who opposed them.

1. Preachers who espoused the cause of abstinence.

Though it is possible to find many writings from those who
sought to inform Christians of what the Bible says about "wine,"
we will look at just a few who were leaders of the tremendous
effort. Lumpkins gives a list of eminent scholars of the 19th century
who believed and wrote that there were two "wines" in the Bible
(fermented and unfermented):

> Adam Clarke, Albert Barnes, Thomas Scott, Ralph
> Wardlaw, F.R. Lees, James Smith, George Duffield,
> Dawson Burns, Taylor Lewis, William Patton, G. W.
> Samson, Moses Stewart, Canon F.W. Farrar, Alonzo
> Potter, G. Bush, and Norman Kerr.[54]

This list is long, but is not complete, as he has not mentioned all who have written. To show their common belief and thesis, we will quote from a very recent book, *Ancient Wine and the Bible*, who attributes the following quote to Dr. Moses Stuart (1780-1852), a Bible Scholar, well-educated and a prolific writer.

> My final conclusion is this, namely, that, whenever
> the Scriptures speak of wine as a comfort, a blessing,
> or a libation to God, and rank it with such articles as
> corn and oil, they can mean, only such wine as con-
> tained no alcohol that could have a mysterious ten-
> dency; that, whenever they denounce it, prohibit
> it, and connect it with drunkenness and reveling,,
> they can mean only alcohol or intoxicaing wine.[55]

The availability of writings from the early 1800's has been greatly helped by the fact that Google has put many of them on the internet in Google Books.

2. Lyman Beecher: Cofounder of the American Temperance Society.

Lyman Beecher was a Presbyterian pastor in Boston in the early 1800's. By 1826 when he began preaching on intemperance, he was known as one of the foremost preachers of his day and his efforts resulted in a significant spiritual awakening. He had a reputation for defending orthodoxy. His messages on alcohol were not particularly appreciated in Boston. In fact, he knew several set-backs, but always persevered. He proposed to his fellow ministers a program for combating intemperance in 1812 but the response was clearly negative:

> ... the regular committee reported that 'after faithful and prayerful inquiry' it was convinced that nothing could be done to check the growth of intemperance.[56]

But he persisted and soon headed another committee which began to print and distribute information towards reducing the consumption of alcohol, especially in religious services. His messages and his work produced results. He co-founded the American Temperance Society in 1826, and that society grew quickly. His "Six Sermons on Intemperance," given in 1828, gave powerful support for temperance. His message was simple.

> Intemperance is the sin of our land, and if anything shall defeat the hopes of the world, which hang upon our experiment of civil liberty, it is that river of fire [intemperance], which is rolling through the land, destroying the vital air, and extending around an atmosphere of death.[57]

This message was sorely needed, for the liquor industry was booming. By 1810, whiskey and other distilled liquors constituted the country's third most important industrial product, and distilling was a notable economic activity on the frontier because of the high costs of shipping grain. The price of alcoholic products dropped significantly and the number of those that indulged rose steeply.

Within five years there were 2,220 local chapters of the Temperance Society in the US with 170,000 members who had taken a pledge to abstain from drinking distilled beverages.[58] Beecher later moved from Boston to Cincinnati where he continued his preaching on the subject.

3. George Marshall: Noted Jurist and Converted Alcoholic.

George Marshall was a Canadian judge in Nova Scotia. In 1823 he was named chief justice of the Inferior Court of Common Pleas. He also served as president of the Courts of General and Special Sessions and justice of the peace for Cape Breton. He was well known and wrote a definitive work on Canadian Law. In 1824, after a significant time of soul-searching and searching the Scriptures, he accepted the Lord as his personal Savior. He stopped all "partaking" of alcoholic beverages in 1824. He visited Boston in 1831 and read Lyman Beecher's sermons.

In 1842, he retired as a judge and started traveling and speaking against alcohol across Canada, in the United States, and in Great Britain. In 1855 he wrote *Strong Drink Delusion, with its Criminal and Ruinous Results Exposed*, which I found on Microfilm in Laval University in Quebec, Canada. It has now been republished. In this book he documented the case for grape juice in the Bible, both from Scripture and from ancient writings. In a book written in 1866, he details a great many of the crimes he had encountered while on the bench and the influence of alcohol in those crimes, saying:

> ... all through my judicial experience, I found,-as has been the same with every Judge,-that the great proportion of crimes, of every degree, with which I had to deal, were more or less attributable to the use of intoxicating drink.[59]

4. Eliphalet Nott: Noted Pastor, Scientist, Inventor, College President.

Eliphalet Nott was one of the most respected pastors, scholars, and lecturers of his time. He was also a scientist with several noted inventions, including the first anthracite coal stove, which was named for him. In 1798, he became pastor of the First Presbyterian Church of Albany, New York, which included a number of prestigious political leaders in the congregation.

In 1800 he was named co-chaplain of the New York State legislature and a trustee of Union College in Schenectady. In 1804 he was named president of that college which was the third largest in America, behind Yale and Harvard. Under Nott's presidency, Union College flourished and graduated the largest class in the United States at that time. His most famous series of lectures was "Lectures on Temperance" published in 1847. He was a fiery advocate of abstinence and regularly declared that the Bible could not be used to defend moderate drinking:

> In the preceding lectures, we have shown that a kind of wine has existed from great antiquity, which was injurious to health and subversive of morals; that these evils, since the introduction of distillation, have been greatly increased; that half the lunacy, three-fourths of the pauperism, and five-sixths of the crime with which the nation is visited, is owing to intemperance;

> ...as far as the wines of commerce are concerned, to appeal to the Bible as authority [for consuming them], is absurd [for the] Bible knows nothing and teaches nothing directly, in relation to these wines of commerce-the same being either a brandied

> or drugged article, never in use in Palestine; that
> in relation to these spurious articles the book of
> nature must alone be consulted, and that being
> consulted, their condemnation will be found on
> many a page, inscribed in characters of wrath...[60]

Doctor Nott was very well educated, and he used the fiery language of his time. I have read many statements that are frankly contemptuous of those who wrote in the early 1800's. It is disgraceful that we should dismiss their findings so easily when they were very godly men who studied the subject meticulously. It should be noted that there were a great many such men.

5. Opposition to Abstinence from Preachers.

In the battle for abstinence it is not to be thought that those who so ably espoused abstinence from a biblical standpoint did not face vigorous opposition from those who denigrated their position. Most of the clergy in denominations that were turning liberal partook freely of alcoholic beverages and were firmly opposed to any thought that the Bible did *not* condone moderate drinking. This opposition was very outspoken.

One of the most vocal was Howard Crosby, pastor of Fourth Avenue Presbyterian Church, New York City, and Chancellor of New York University beginning in 1870. When invited to speak in the pulpit of a noted proponent of total abstinence, he gave a discourse which he entitled "Calm View of the Temperance Question." In his address, he asserts that the total abstinence system is contrary to revealed religion and harmful to the interests of the country, exclaiming:

> I charge upon this system [total abstinence] the
> growth of drunkenness in our land and the general

demoralization among religious communities; and I call upon all sound-minded thinking men to stop the enormities of this false system.[61]

Later he wrote,

There is not a chemist or a classical scholar in the world who would dare risk his reputation on the assertion that there was ever an unfermented wine in common use [in Bible times], knowing well, that "must" preserved from fermentation is called wine only by a kind of courtesy... and that this could never, in the nature of things be a common drink.[62]

Prof. Burnstead makes similar assertions; declaring that the "theory" of an unfermented wine has failed to commend itself to the scholarship of the world.[63]

Dr. Moore, a contemporary of Dr. Crosby, remarked, "The history of the doctrine of unfermented Bible wine cannot be carried back beyond a few decades; and this fact furnishes a "préjugé légitime" against it (a legitimate prejudice)."[64] He is saying that the lack of longevity of the "unfermented Bible wine" doctrine is a sufficient reason for not believing that theory. This can also be seen in another quote from an author in 1883:

At the opening of the present year, [1881] and almost simultaneously, Chancellor Crosby on the platform of the Monday Lectureship, Dr. Moore in the pages of the "Presbyterian Review," and Prof. Burnstead in the pages of the " Bibliotheca Sacra," made vigorous onslaught on those who hold that the Bible does not lend its sanction to the use of intoxicating beverages, and, in particular, on all who quote the example of Christ in favor of total abstinence.[65]

Chancellor Crosby was a spirited and contemptuous foe of the temperance movement. He said that there is a class of biblical scholars and interpreters "who do assert that wherever wine is referred to in the Bible with approbation it is unfermented wine." Of this class of men, Dr. Crosby says:

> "their learned ignorance is splendid"; they are "inventors of a theory of magnificent daring"; they "use false texts" and "deceptive arguments"; "deal dishonestly with the Scriptures"; "beg the question and build on air"; their theory is a "fable," born of "falsehoods," supported by "Scripture-twisting and wriggling"; their arguments are "cobwebs," and their zeal outstrips their judgment, and they plan to "undermine the Bible."[66]

More than one hundred years later, many modern writers and speakers who promote moderate drinking also seem to convey the thought that grape juice in the Bible is a fairly new idea in the Christian community and is promoted by unworthy and dishonest writers. Nothing could be further from the truth. The dates and the quotes already furnished in this chapter prove that very proficient and respected students of God's Word taught, preached, and wrote about grape juice in the Bible in preceding centuries.

It is interesting to compare those who espouse the cause of abstinence with those of the 1800s who opposed them. On the one hand there was scholarship, searching ancient texts and studying the biblical references to try to understand the text. On the other hand, it is observed that in the 1800's there was character assassination of and ridicule toward those who found "grape juice" in the Bible. Those who reject grape juice in the Bible today do not have a very flattering opinion of those who accept this truth either; historically, that has always been the case.

VIII. CAN WE EVEN KNOW WHAT IS TRUE?

T he title of this book could very well have been: *Grape Juice Is in the Bible: True or False?* for the task of this study is to determine "what is the Truth of the matter." Unfortunately, we are living in an era when, even among theologians, there is considerable debate as to whether or not objective truth exists and if it is possible to know what truth is.

That there should be such a debate is sad! To say that the Creator of the universe does not know what truth is or how to reveal it is sheer unbelief in the God of the Bible. Can God speak anything but the truth?

There is an interesting article in the magazine, *Israel My Glory*,

> Truth is defined as that which conforms to reality. Not reality as people think they see it, but reality as it actually exists-as only God sees it. For the God-breathed Scriptures to be anything less than the truth, God must have made a mistake or lied.[67]

Truth is certainly important to God. He uses words like truth and true and truly almost 400 times in the Bible. Renald Showers says the following:

> The Scriptures repeatedly associate what is true and truth with God. The primary Old Testament word used for this association is "emet" (Hebrew). Its foundational concept is "certainty, dependability";

> and it is used "in several categories of contexts, all
> of which relate to God directly or indirectly."[68]

From this and many Scripture passages, it can be affirmed that:
- Biblical Truth is absolute, never relative.
- Biblical Truth is objective, never subjective.
- Biblical Truth is what corresponds to reality.
- Biblical Truth must always be consistent-God cannot announce two conflicting truths.
- Biblical Truth is said to be eternal. It does not change.

God's Word says in Deuteronomy 32:4, "He is the Rock, his work is perfect: for all his ways are judgment: a God of truth and without iniquity, just and right is he." David says, "Lead me in thy truth, and teach me: for thou art the God of my salvation; on thee do I wait all the day" (Ps. 25:5). The Psalmist goes further: "God, Which made heaven, and earth, the sea, and all that therein is, which keepeth truth forever." Finally, Jesus said, "I am the truth."

In today's culture, the increasingly popular conception of truth makes it subject to human experience. This idea simply rejects the plain sense of Scripture. The truth of Scripture is objective, not subjective, and is never affected by the interpreter's understanding or lack of understanding of Biblical truth.

It is a fact that Christians in America are less and less interested in "objective truth." In fact, there has been a massive swing away from truth as truth, as affirmed by the results of a poll published by World Magazine, Aug. 2008, pp. 4 and 26:

- 63% of Americans don't think that truth is knowable.
- 53% of those who call themselves evangelical Christians are similarly skeptical.
- Most Americans agree that there are clear and absolute standards for what is right and wrong. But a little more

than half rely on "practical experience and common sense." Only 29 % say that their religion is their guide for determining those standards.

Raymond Teachout, a Baptist missionary in French Guiana, has written a book, *Adrift from the Gospel*, which speaks much about *"truth."* He says in discussing the *"interpretation barrier"*:

> Few Evangelicals put in question the fact that God has given us His revelation. However, what is often put in question is the clarity and perspicuity of Scripture. "Yes," they would say, "truth has been given. But it is beyond us to ever come to a sure interpretation of that revealed truth."[69]

Consider this quote from John Stott. He says in his popular book, *Evangelical Truth*:

> In particular, we need a greater measure of discernment, so that we may distinguish between evangelical essentials which cannot be compromised and those adiaphora (matters indifferent) on which being of secondary importance it is not necessary for us to insist.
>
> ...Whenever equally biblical Christians, who are equally anxious to understand the teaching of Scripture and to submit to its authority, reach different conclusions, we should deduce that evidently, Scripture is not crystal clear in this matter, and therefore we can afford to give one another liberty.[70]

He is effectively saying, "If everybody doesn't agree on a passage of Scripture, it is because the text is not clear." Raymond Teachout goes on to say of such an idea: "In calling into question the clarity and/or sufficiency of Scripture, it is impossible to come to a sure interpretation of Scripture."[71]

In other words, if one does not accept the principle of the clarity and/or sufficiency of Scripture, one cannot understand Scripture! It must be added here that the fact that God's Revelation is clear-meant to be understood-is one of the basic rules of biblical interpretation which goes back to the time of the Reformation and which will be discussed in the next chapter.

There are two passages of Scripture that sum this up clearly and explain why Scripture is clear to some, but not to others. Simply put, those who *believe* in what God has said, or who have faith in His revelation, can know and understand what He has revealed. Hebrews 11:3 says, "Through faith we understand that the worlds were framed by the Word of God, so that things which are seen were not made of things which do appear." Paul says in Romans 1:20, "For the invisible things of him from the creation of the world are clearly seen, being understood by the things that are made, even his eternal power and Godhead …"

In the diagram at the right we realize that only God's Revelation enables humanity to

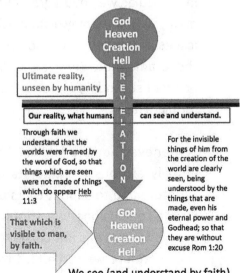

We see (and understand by faith) through a glass, darkly I Cor 13:12.

66

perceive truths that are clearly evident in God's reality-if we believe His Revelation.

In the search for the truth concerning the reality of fresh grape juice in the Bible, the thesis that the Word of God is not clear and is therefore open to diverse ways of interpreting a given Scripture, would make it impossible to know the truth. Yet the Bible, in Jesus' own words, says: "And ye shall know the truth, and the truth shall make you free" (John 8:32). It is obvious that if God's truth does not express reality, it will certainly not make us free. And it is equally obvious that if we cannot understand it, it will still not make us free.

But Jesus' words are true, and we can have confident assurance that one can know the truth of the Bible. This is supported by a great many other passages in the Bible.

There follows here a quote from "Adrift from the Gospel" which will help us in the study of the principles of interpretation of the Bible in the next chapter. This discussion illustrates the fact that in the Bible:

1. The truth has been revealed,
2. The truth is understandable, and
3 The solution to understanding Scriptural truth is humility and faithfulness.[72]

1. The Truth Has Been Revealed (Jn. 18:38; Heb. 11:1, 6-7).

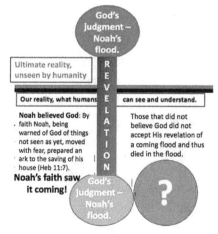

The story of Noah will serve as a good model. The reality of judgment (the flood) was revealed by God to Noah, who believed the revelation, understood the plain sense of it, and then acted upon it. Noah made known this revelation as a preacher of righteousness (2 Pet. 2:5), but no one other than his family would believe. All the other people preferred thinking that there would not be a flood and they perished in terror.

For us also, if we do not accept God's revelation, we would be blocked, unable to know that which is the ultimate reality and end of all things, and we would perish in our sins.

However, God has revealed the truth (Heb. 1:1; 2:1-3; 2 Tim. 3:15-17; Ps. 19; Rom. 1:18-19). Like Noah, it is both possible and necessary that we align our beliefs and faith with what God reveals as to the ultimate reality of things. By faith, it is necessary to accept the revealed warning of judgment and offer of salvation in Jesus Christ.

2. The Truth Is Understandable

Not only did God reveal truth, but He revealed it in a way for it to be understood. In fact, God made the truth understandable to the point of making man accountable to that revelation. Man is without excuse because God has made known the truth (c.f. John 12:47-48). Paul's epistle to Titus develops the subject of the importance of truth. That is why Paul exhorts Titus to proclaim with authority the Word of God (Tit. 1:9; 2:15).

Unfortunately, some would argue that we have no real basis of truly knowing, because we cannot be sure to have

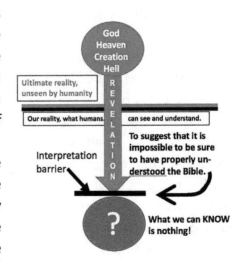

properly understood God's Revelation. An interpretation barrier of some sort is set up by that argument, barring us from the certainty of knowing the truth (i.e. we are only able to think we know the truth; we are confined to the realm of opinions...). This is sometimes what motivates people to be inclusive in their outlook, that is to say, to accept many opposing interpretations.

What does the Bible say regarding the problem of interpretation? 2 Peter 3:14-16 mentions that some parts of Scripture are hard to understand, but in saying "hard" it does not mean impossible. If even the hard parts of Scripture are able to be understood, how much more the parts that define fundamentally what is a true Christian? In fact, Peter warns in that passage about those who twist the meaning of Scripture unto their own ruin.

In Mark 12:24, Christ's reaction to those who questioned him was not: "Oh, I see how the Bible was not clear on that subject..." (God forbid!). It was rather: "Do ye not therefore err, because ye know not the scriptures, neither the power of God?"

Man gets all the blame for misunderstanding the Bible, for the Bible, in itself is clear in what it reveals. Man's deceitful heart is the source of the problem. There is no such thing as an interpretation barrier.

3. Solution: Humility and Faithfulness

The proper response to God's model of revelation is not flippant and superficial dictatorial arrogance (as we sometimes sadly see), but a serious study of God's Word in order to be able to be found as "workman that needeth not to be ashamed, rightly dividing the Word of God" (2 Tim. 2:15). 1Thessalonians 5:21-22 says: "Prove all things, hold fast that which is good."

We must proclaim what God says faithfully, without adding to it, or taking away from it (Prov. 30:5-6; 2 Tim. 4:1-2; Tit. 2:1, 15).

The unsaved will be judged according to the Word of God at the great white throne (Rev. 20:11-15; John 12:48; Rom. 2:16). Christians will give account unto God at Christ's judgment seat (2 Cor. 4:5; 5:10). Those who preach and teach God's Word will be judged more severely (James 3:1). It is not because no one will be perfectly faithful that one should not strive for that faithfulness God desires of us. (Here ends the quote from "Adrift from the Gospel".)

It is certain that if the ancient words from God in the Bible do not express truth, then they are not from God and can do nothing for us.

But they do express truth-truth that is knowable, understandable, absolute, objective, and which corresponds to reality. Truth, according to the *Theological Dictionary of the New Testament*, "is used absolutely to denote a reality which is to be regarded as 'firm,' and therefore 'solid,' 'valid,' or 'binding.' "[73] In the present study, it will be found that the truth of the matter is that there is indeed grape juice in the Bible. This truth will then help us to know what God wants us to do as Christians about alcoholic consumption.

IX. RIGHTLY DIVIDING THE WORD OF TRUTH

As I was researching the question of what the Bible says about grape juice, I had an interview with one of the leading opponents of the "grape juice in the Bible" position. He has a PhD and teaches, among other subjects, biblical hermeneutics, which is the study of the theory and practice of the interpretation of the Bible. He kept saying that there was no mention of grape juice in the Bible, and I kept citing verses to show that there was indeed mention of grape juice. Finally, he said: "It is simply a matter of hermeneutics." I agreed with him immediately on that statement, though I disagree strongly with his interpretation. For example, by stringing Scriptures together you can understand the following "false truth": "Judas went out and hanged himself, Go thou and do likewise." Both parts of this "instruction" are from the Bible, but not in the same context. In fact, they are not even in the same section or book of the Bible:

> Judas Iscariot, one of the twelve, went unto the chief priests, to betray him unto them. When he saw that he was condemned, repented himself, and brought again the thirty pieces of silver to the chief priests and elders, Saying, I have sinned. And he cast down the pieces of silver in the temple, and departed, and went and hanged himself (Mark 14:10). Go, and do thou likewise (Luke 10:37).

The Bible does not teach that as a result of sinning, the solution is hanging oneself. The sentences strung together above do not represent Scriptural truth. There is no respect for the context of each phrase. Though the words come from Scripture, the paragraph as it is thus written, is not God's truth.

God's Word is a complete written revelation, His perfect and clear communication to man. Let's look at what He says:

> O LORD, thou art my God; I will exalt thee, I will praise thy name; for thou hast done wonderful things; thy counsels of old are faithfulness and truth (Isa. 25:1).

> For the word of the LORD is right; and all his works are done in truth (Ps. 33:4).

> For the LORD is good; his mercy is everlasting; and his truth endureth to all generations (Ps. 100:5).

In these verses and in many others in the Bible, we find that God communicated with all generations, not just with those who originally received the revelation. Remember: "whatsoever things were written aforetime were written for our learning." We also find that truth is important to God. In Exodus 34, where God is revealing Himself to Moses, He says this: "The LORD, The LORD God, merciful and gracious, longsuffering, and abundant in goodness and truth" (v. 6.). In one of his most important pronouncements Jesus said, "I am the way, the truth, and the life."

What is truth? Pilate asked that question of Jesus, and it is still an important question today, because in every strata of society "truth" is being attacked. In the modern era, many philosophers and theologians deny the existence of objective reality or truth, saying: "Reality is in the mind of the beholder" or "We create our own truth." It should not surprise us that everyone has begun to doubt the fact of truth. Dr. Dave Miller says:

Perhaps the greatest deterrent to a proper interpretation of the Bible is the widespread and
growing sense of uncertainty in the acquisition of
absolute truth. American civilization has been inun-
dated with pluralism and has been brow-beaten
into accepting the notion that one belief is as good
as another and that it really does not matter what
one believes. [74]

In this study, we will follow the historical definition of truth,
given above: "Truth is defined as that which conforms to reality."

What then is our responsibility? It is to seek truth in God's
Word, to endeavor to understand it, and to apply it in our lives.
David said, "O my God, I trust in thee... Lead me in thy truth and
teach me: for thou art the God of my salvation; on thee do I wait
all the day" (Ps. 25:2, 5). David had a tremendous respect for truth
for he mentioned it often in the Psalms and he actively sought it
from God. He says in Psalms 119:94, "I am thine, save me; for I
have sought thy precepts."

Is it possible to misunderstand God's truth, what He has said in
His Word? Very definitely. Even Bible scholars can misunderstand
words, thoughts, and teaching from the Bible. Jesus' disciples spent
three and a half years listening to Him, the greatest teacher that
ever lived, and yet they misunderstood Him at least twice. Jesus
met two of his disciples on the road to Emmaus and questioned
them as to what they were talking about and why they were sad.
They related to Him the recent events at Jerusalem saying,

The chief priests and our rulers delivered him to be
condemned to death and have crucified him. But
we trusted that it had been he which should have
redeemed Israel ... (Luke 24:20, 21).

73

A literal translation of verse 21 gives: *But we had hoped that he was the one to redeem Israel.*[75] Literally, this means their hope was now dead. It also means that they did not believe that the resurrection had taken place or could take place. Jesus was dead and all hope of the Kingdom was gone. It was evident that they had not understood the teaching of Jesus when He foretold His death and resurrection from the grave. He had clearly spoken on the issue several times and He had talked of it often in the hours leading up to the event. He had spoken the truth and they did not understand it even though they were face to face with Him and there was no problem of language or culture. They were hindered by their preconceived belief that His Kingdom was to come immediately.

A second occurrence of a clear misunderstanding of Jesus' teaching is found in Acts 1:6, "When they therefore were come together, they asked of him, saying, Lord, wilt thou at this time restore again the kingdom to Israel?"

The disciples were expecting Him to chase out the Romans and to install His Kingdom immediately. Even though Jesus had never taught this, it was often in their thoughts. Though their thoughts had been turned completely upside down by His death, with the miraculous, supernatural fact of the resurrection, their expectation of a soon-to-be kingdom had resurfaced. However, in His teaching, Jesus had spoken to them many times of His plan for the immediate future and these plans did not include setting up His Kingdom on earth at that time. He was preparing them for a ministry that would take place after His return to Heaven. He had said "My kingdom is not of this world" and "I go unto my father" and "I go to prepare a place for you." His discussion with Peter in John 21 concerned that which Peter and John would do after His departure and before His return. And yet, they still did not understand what He had said-they still asked Him in Acts 1:6, "Wilt thou at this time restore again the kingdom to Israel?" Though Daniel had clearly spoken of this over 400 years before, they did not understand that there would be a delay in the establishment of the Kingdom. We can understand why they did not put all this together in their minds: these instances are mentioned here only to show that it is possible to misunderstand even divine truth.

So, what can we do today, almost two thousand years later? We must diligently seek to fully understand God's Word, respecting the miraculous nature of it and realizing that there are some special considerations for proper understanding of it.

First, we need to define "interpretation." The popular meaning is "to find your own meaning for something." The biblical meaning is "to unfold the meaning of what is said, to explain, to expound." A perfect example of this is Jesus' response to His disciples' misunderstanding on the road to Emmaus:

> O fools, and slow of heart to believe all that the prophets have spoken:... And beginning at Moses and all the prophets, he "expounded" unto them in all the scriptures the things concerning himself. Luke 24:25, 27.

Jesus' method of interpreting the truth about Himself was to give the entire context of God's Revelation concerning Himself.

Secondly, in order to interpret a word or passage correctly, we must consider the following statement: "If God has caused His message to be recorded in the Bible for mankind, then we would expect Him to use human communication that is simple and understandable" (i.e., propositional truth expressed in human language). Therefore, when we interpret the Bible, we must approach it as if it is God's plain word to us, spoken through His prophets in time-space history. It is to be taken literally and accepted completely unless the context indicates otherwise. Years ago, my hermeneutics professor in Bible school summed up the practice of interpretation this way: "If the plain sense makes good sense, seek no other sense."

Thirdly, we must consider the context of a word or passage. What is "context"?

1. The circumstances that form the setting for an event, statement, or idea, and in terms of which it can be fully understood and assessed.
2. The parts of something written or spoken that immediately precede and follow a word or passage and clarify its meaning.[76]

Guy duty wrote a book which listed eight rules of [Bible] interpretation. One of these was the following:

> The rule of context: The meaning must be gathered from the context. Every word you read must be understood in the light of the words that come before and after it. Many passages will not be understood at all, or understood incorrectly, without the help afforded by the context.[77]

When this rule is not respected, when Bible words are used out of context, one can prove almost anything. Some interpreters twist them from a natural to a non-natural sense.

In biblical interpretation there are several contexts, and they must all be respected: grammatical, historical, theological, and Christological. We must

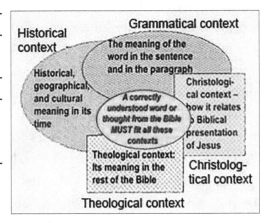

understand not only the meaning of the word or phrase in the sentence or paragraph but also the meaning in the historical culture when it was written and the meaning in relation to other biblical teaching which concerns it. Careful attention should be given to its meaning, especially as it touches the teaching about Jesus. Just as a puzzle piece must fit all the sides which touch it, so the correct meaning will make sense when all the contexts that concern it agree.

Let's look at grammatical context. Words are grouped into sentences, paragraphs, and chapters for communication. They must be understood as they relate between themselves and this relation is called context. Consider an example from Scripture:

> And in the vine were three branches: and it was
> as though it budded, and her blossoms shot forth;
> and the clusters thereof brought forth ripe grapes:
> And Pharaoh's cup was in my hand: and I took the
> grapes, and pressed them into Pharaoh's cup, and
> I gave the cup into Pharaoh's hand (Gen. 40:10, 11).

That which was squeezed into Pharaoh's cup was quite certainly grape juice, from the context (surrounding phrases). It would be foolish to understand anything else. The butler took "grapes" and "squeezed" them. The result can only be grape juice, not fermented wine. Here is the solution for those who accept the proper interpretation of this story. Even though our English Bibles call the product of this squeezing "wine," it was fresh, without alcohol. Josephus, an educated 1st century Jewish historian, told the story of Pharaoh's cup and called this product *"oinos"* or wine. The Greek word *oinos* was a generic word in Josephus' time which could mean either an alcoholic beverage, or fresh grape juice, depending on the context.

Another example of respecting the context of written words is the biblical word, *"winepress."* This word was used historically to describe an enclosure in which grapes were put to be trampled so that the juice could run out and be captured. The Bible speaks of "the fulness of the winepress" (Num. 18:27) and "the increase of the winepress" (Num. 18:30). This fullness or increase can only mean fresh grape juice as it was the first product of the crushed raw material, grapes. Therefore, a "wine press" was actually a "grape press." We see that the historical context is vital here.

I repeat again for emphasis: Just as a puzzle piece must fit *all* the sides which touch it, so the correct meaning will make sense when *all* the contexts that concern it agree. When all the facts of an interpretation are in agreement they sound together in harmony, like notes in a chord.

Besides this basic rule of respecting the context, thoughtful Bible scholars have developed certain special rules down through the centuries that help interpret Scripture. This is because it must be interpreted differently than other ancient writings as it is a supernatural book. These rules of biblical interpretation will be listed here and briefly applied in the study of grape juice in the Bible.

1. God's WORD is spiritually discerned; you must be born again to understand it.

This is simple, logical, and biblical. If a person has not accepted God's gift of salvation which is provided as a result of believing in Christ's sacrificial death on the cross, he cannot understand God's Revelation.

> But the natural man receiveth not the things of the
> Spirit of God: for they are foolishness unto him:

neither can he know them, because they are spiri-
tually discerned, (1 Cor. 2:14).

It was Calvin who noted-and the apostle Paul who stated in 1 Corinthians 2:14-15-that the Word of God is *spiritual*, and, there-fore, can only be perceived and discerned by the spiritual man. Ramm says:

> The first spiritual qualification of the interpreter
> is *that he be born again.* Angus and Green write,
> "This first principle of Biblical interpretation is taken
> from the Bible itself."... The final spiritual qualifica-
> tion is that of *utter dependence on the Holy Spirit
> to guide and direct.* [78]

There is a tremendous amount of discussion on the internet concerning the subject of grape juice in the Bible. Many of those who "post" on the internet make no pretense of being born again nor do they accept God's word as being inspired truth. And yet some of these "experts" are quoted by Christian writers in dis-cussing "wine" in the Bible. We should not consult such experts, much less accept their conclusions, especially as to what Jesus created and drank.

2. God's WORD is God-given-inspired, inerrant, and pre-served for us.

The Bible is not a book that we can approach as other ancient writings, where we can make the author say what seems sen-sible to us.

> All Scripture is given by inspiration of God... For the
> prophecy came not in old time by the will of man:

but holy men of God spake as they were moved
by the Holy Ghost. For whatsoever things were
written aforetime were written for our learning,
that we through patience and comfort of the scriptures might have hope. (2 Tim. 3:16, 2 Pet. 1:21,
Rom. 15:4.)

These excerpts from the verses mean that the Bible was
written in ancient times by men who were so controlled by God
that what they wrote was exactly what God wanted them to
write. This means also that God did not make any mistakes in the
Bible in the original autographs, even in the words that He used.
Jesus authenticated all the Hebrew letters that composed the Old
Testament: "I say unto you, Till heaven and earth pass, one jot
or one tittle shall in no wise pass from the law" (Matt. 5:18). He
was referring, not just to the words, but to the *letters* of Scripture.
We can never say that God used the wrong word in the Bible. We
must not find our own logical meaning to a biblical word or phrase,
but only try to understand what He meant by the words He used.
Andrew Kulikovsky says:

The doctrine of Biblical Inspiration is fundamental
to evangelical Christianity. Without this essential
notion, the uniqueness and authority of the Bible
is destroyed. The Bible just becomes one of many
ancient books and the truths of historic Christianity
are reduced to a collection of religious myths.[79]

3. God's WORD is progressive-it builds from the account
   of the creation to the prophecies of Revelation.

Heb 1:1, 2 says: "God, who at sundry times and in divers man-
ners spake in time past unto the fathers by the prophets, Hath

in these last days spoken unto us by his Son ..." The sense of this verse is that God spoke in the past and spoke more fully by His Son after the Incarnation. We had better understand Jesus' words here because it is superior to God's Revelation that was given prior to Jesus' coming.

This brings us to understand the principle that God's Revelation to man was *progressive*, God did not reveal all of it at once, but to many men over the space of more than 1100 years. Without going into details about the different historical situations in which God spoke to man, we will simply affirm that each man already possessed the Revelation that God had given before him. Thus, Abraham understood more of what God said to him than Noah would have, and Paul understood a great deal more than Moses, because much more of God's revelation was available to him. Of course, we can understand infinitely more than the Jews who listened to Jesus, because we have the entire New Testament to add to the Old. Accepting this principle of Biblical Interpretation is vital to understanding Scripture.

> There is a definite progression in Scripture, and unless this principle of progress is recognized there can be no clear exegesis of Scripture. Progressive revelation means that as the timeline of history unravels, the plan and purpose of God becomes fuller and clearer; the meat is slowly being put on the bones, if you will.[80]

4. God's WORD is one complete Revelation-God is the author of all of it and His written Word is what He has to say to us.

We must never forget that in the Bible, it is always God who is speaking. He simply cannot say something in one part of Scripture that contradicts what He has said in another part of Scripture. He must be consistent. The Bible covers centuries of time. For instance, there are over five hundred years between Moses' writings and the book of Isaiah. God, the author of all Scripture, knew what He had said before Isaiah wrote by inspiration, and He meant His truth to continue until our time and beyond. "For the LORD is good; his mercy is everlasting; and his truth endureth to all generations" (Ps. 100:5). We affirm that the words and truths that He uses in one part of Scripture must agree with everything He has said in all of Scripture, for He must always be consistent.

This fourth rule of Bible Interpretation is taught clearly in the Bible by two words: *all* and *Scripture*. It is "all Scripture" that is given by inspiration of God, which is profitable to correct us and teach us God's way. Jesus corrected the thinking of the two disciples on the road to Emmaus by going back through all Scripture and He used those two words in His teaching: "beginning at Moses and all the prophets, he expounded unto them in all the scriptures the things concerning himself" (Luke 24:27). Scripture is the translation of the Greek word for writing. Geisler says:

> The New Testament uses the term 'Scripture' in a technical sense. It occurs some fifty times, and in most cases, it refers unmistakably to the Old Testament as a whole. To first-century Christians, the word 'Scripture' meant primarily the canon of the Old Testament, which is called "sacred" (2 Tim. 3:15) or "holy" (Rom. 1:2).[81]

Jesus clearly emphasized the importance of *all Scripture*. He spoke often about an act or a word saying that it happened in order that Scripture *might be fulfilled*. This was even more important as His death approached for He used the entire phrase "in order that Scripture might be fulfilled" three times in John 17 and 19.

(The phrase was used twenty-one times in the Bible, each time to signify something that happened to fulfill God's spoken and written Word).

Another Scriptural word that describes God's perfect consistency throughout His entire Revelation is *"faithful"*: "Know therefore that the LORD thy God, he is God, the faithful God, which keepeth covenant," (Deut. 7:9). George Denise says, "To affirm that God is consistent means He never becomes greater, better, or worse; He never learns, grows, develops, improves, evolves, or gets younger or older."[82] *The Complete Topical Guide to the Bible* goes further: "God's nature, plans and actions do not change even though he is active and his relationships do not remain static. His moral consistency guarantees his commitment to unchanging principles."[83]

In our interpretation of the biblical word "wine", we must find an understanding that must work in every single case. This is clearly not the case in the current popular understanding that "wine" in the Bible always means an alcoholic beverage.

An example of this is the illustration given by Jesus in three passages (Mark 2:22, Matt. 9:17, and Luke 5:37–39): "not putting new wine in old wineskins, lest the wine ferment and break the wineskins." The usual interpretation that is given to this is new wine that begins to ferment would burst the wineskin. Brumbelow treats this passage in his chapter on "controversial passages in the Bible that deal with wine." He says that, "this was not the point at all" and goes on to say, "New wine that began to ferment would burst new or old wineskins." This fact was recognized by Job centuries earlier: "Behold, my belly is as wine which hath no vent; it is ready to burst like new bottles" (Job 32:19). Brumbelow says further:

> The point was to prevent fermentation. The
> yeast/leaven from old wine skins could infect and

cause new wine, sweet wine to ferment and spoil. Cleanliness was crucial in preserving new wine {grape juice}. Luke mentions, "and both {the wine skin and the wine} are preserved" Luke 5:38. The new wine is preserved in that state of being unfermented and the new wineskin is preserved. It should also be noted that Jesus himself is calling "wine" that which is unfermented.

Jerome, commenting on Matthew 9:17, says that "new skins, must be used for wine that is to be preserved as 'must', because the remains of former ferment and attaches to old skins." G. W. Sampson informs us of "The Roman custom of using new flasks in preparing and preserving wines permanently unfermented, lest the remains of ferment adhering to the inside of an old wine-flask should cause ferment in the corked and sealed must." Ernest Gordon concludes that Christ's few references to wine are easily understood.[84]

This message of the proper understanding of new wine in old wineskins depends upon the proper meaning of "wine" throughout the entire Bible.

5. God's WORD is clear-meant to be understood.

God says in Isaiah 45:19, "I have not spoken in secret, in a dark place of the earth: I said not unto the seed of Jacob, Seek ye me in vain: I the LORD speak righteousness [what is just, normal, or true], I declare things that are right." This is a very important principle. Bernard Ramm said: "The Bible was given to us in the form of human language and therefore appeals to human reason-it invites investigation."[85] Martin Luther believed that, in a physical sense, one could clearly understand the plain teaching of Scripture in applying regular rules of grammar and hermeneutics to the text of Scripture. He added that there was always a spiritual sense in which the believer is aided by the illumination of the Holy Spirit.

Not only did God give His revelation to be understood, but He also interprets it for us! The following quote is from Ramm's book on Biblical Interpretation:

> Around the time of the Reformation, the Roman Catholic Church insisted that it was 'gifted with the grace of interpretation,' and therefore, it knew instinctively the interpretation of Scripture. The Reformers rejected this erroneous claim and set in its place the rule that Scripture is its own inter-preter-"Scriptura sacra sui ipsius interpres ..." What it means, very simply, is that the Bible as a whole interprets the various parts, and hence no single aspect of the Word can be so interpreted as to destroy the teaching of the whole.[86]

This very basic rule of Biblical Interpretation simply reinforces the application of the preceding hermeneutical rules that we have applied to the understanding of grape juice in the Bible. God never contradicts Himself. When we consult two biblical passages on the same subject, proper interpretation helps us to come to a full understanding of both.

In Nehemiah 10:37, the order is given to "bring the first fruits of our dough, and our offerings, and the fruit of all manner of trees, of wine and of oil, unto the priests, to the chambers of the house of our God ..."

This verse is especially interesting. It tells the Jews to bring "wine" to the priests, into the house of God. But there is a seeming contradiction here with another Scripture for, according to Leviticus 10:9, God gave a command to the priests which carried with it a severe punishment if broken:

> Do not drink wine nor strong drink, thou, nor thy
> sons with thee, when ye go into the tabernacle of
> the congregation, lest ye die: it shall be a statute
> forever throughout your generations.

Ezekiel repeats this prohibition in 44:21: "Neither shall any priest drink wine, when they enter into the inner court." This contradicts all of the passages in the Bible that speak of "drink offerings." These are mentioned thirty-eight times, with Numbers 28:14 specifying: "And their drink offerings shall be half an hin of wine unto a bullock, and the third part of an hin unto a ram, and a fourth part of an hin unto a lamb: this is the burnt offering of every month throughout the months of the year." And yet, Nehemiah 10:37 records the instruction: "... we should bring the first-fruits of our dough, and our offerings, and the fruit of all manner of trees, of wine and of oil, unto the priests, to the chambers of the house of our God ..." God would seem to say in the two passages: "Priests must not drink wine in the temple" and "you must bring wine into the temple for the priests." Since God is always consistent and cannot contradict Himself, we must understand that He is talking here about two different wines: the "wine" in Leviticus and Ezekiel must be fermented and the *wine* in Nehemiah must be grape juice! In the case of Nehemiah's order to bring the wine into the temple, we are helped to understand by the fact that the Hebrew word for wine in this place is *tirosh* which means literally "unfermented grape juice."

There are, of course, a great many other examples of God's Word interpreting itself and making things clear for us. There is a particular question which is often raised today: How can God mislead us concerning the truths about fermented wine in the Bible if the word in our English Bible does not give a clear sense? The answer is to study God's Word-all of God's Word. Paul says, "Study to shew thyself approved unto God, a workman that needeth not to be ashamed, rightly dividing the word of truth" (2 Tim. 2:15). When we consider the added meaning that comes from the Greek, we have: "Study diligently to shew thyself approved unto God, a workman that needeth not to be ashamed, rightly dividing (to cut straight, to proceed on straight paths, hold a straight course, to handle aright, to teach the truth directly and correctly) the word of truth." The Bible was not written in English. The right meaning of each word in our English Bibles must reflect the meaning of the original that was written in Hebrew or Greek.

6. God's WORD has one principal subject-Jesus Christ.

In the Old Testament, Jesus is the promised Messiah from Genesis to Malachi. In the Gospels, Jesus is *"Emmanuel"* or God with us and "the Lamb of God, which taketh away the sin of the world." In the rest of the New Testament, Jesus and His coming are preached and taught.

Paul "preached unto them Jesus, and the resurrection" (Acts 17:18). It is absolutely vital that this rule of Bible Interpretation be respected. The *Chicago Statement on Biblical Hermeneutics, Article III,* puts it this way:

> We affirm that the Person and work of Jesus Christ
> are the central focus of the entire Bible. WE DENY
> that any method of interpretation which rejects
> or obscures the Christ-centeredness of Scripture
> is correct.

> This Affirmation follows the teaching of Christ that
> He is the central theme of Scripture (Matt. 5:17;
> Luke 24:27, 44; John 5:39; Heb. 10:7). This is to say
> that focus on the person and work of Christ runs
> throughout the Bible from Genesis to Revelation.[87]

The life and ministry of Jesus are abundantly narrated in the New Testament, but they are also clearly foretold in the Old Testament, through prophecy as well as pictures and symbols that God used. God revealed to Moses exactly what He wanted in the tabernacle and the sacrifices. The overall message of these symbols is that Jesus is holy and that the Holy One was to be a perfect sacrifice for the sins of His people.

How does this tenet of Biblical Interpretation help us in our study of grape juice? Actually, it is of crucial importance. Let us look at just two events in the life of Christ.

Jesus and the Lord's Supper. The first event that needs to be considered, the Passover Supper, took place just before His death and resurrection. If there is no grape juice in the Bible, then Jesus drank an alcoholic beverage there with His disciples, and He did so against all the typology in the Old Testament. Instead, when He instituted the Lord's Supper for His disciples and for the Church, He partook of what is called in the Greek text, "the fruit of the vine." Since there was grape juice in Bible times, it is very clear that this is that to which He was referring, because the fruit of the vine, or *grape juice*, contained no leaven. Jesus was celebrating the Passover with his disciples and God had very specific commandments for celebrating the Passover. The Pulpit Commentary says: "No leavened bread was to be eaten during that space, and leaven was even to be put away altogether out of all houses."[88] Actually, we must go further and affirm that all sacrifices in the Old Testament prefigured Christ's sacrifice and were "without leaven," which was a type of sin. Leaven (Hebrew, "Chametz") refers to a grain product that is already fermented (i.e., yeast breads, certain types of cake and most alcoholic beverages). The Torah commandments regarding chametz are:

> To remove all chametz from one's home, including things made with chametz, before the first day of Passover. (Ex. 12:15).

> To refrain from eating chametz or mixtures containing chametz during Passover. (Ex. 13:3, Ex. 12:20, Deut. 16:3).

The orthodox Jews to this day make a ceremony of searching out leaven in their homes. Since leaven is a critical component of fermentation, drinking alcoholic wine would violate the Jewish tradition and God's instructions for the Jews. Many Jews, in order to obey God's command, would press out fresh grapes out into cups or pitchers themselves just prior to consumption to make certain that the juice was not fermented.

There can be no doubt as to the presence of yeast in intoxicating wine. Here is an article on making wine by Laurel Gray Vineyards:

> After crushing and pressing, fermentation comes into play. Must (or juice) can begin fermenting naturally within 6–12 hours when aided with wild yeasts in the air. However, many wine makers intervene and add a commercial cultured yeast to ensure consistency and predict the end result.

> Fermentation continues until all of the sugar is converted into alcohol and dry wine is produced. To

create a sweet wine, wine makers will sometimes stop the process before all of the sugar is converted. Fermentation can take anywhere from 10 days to one month or more.[89]

Not only does the interpretation of "the fruit of the vine" as being fermented at the Last Supper cause a problem with the typology of the Passover, but it causes a great problem in looking forward to the Millennial Kingdom. Jesus said, "I will not drink henceforth of this fruit of the vine, until that day when I drink it new with you in my Father's Kingdom" (Matt. 26:26). If this is not grape juice, it would seem that alcohol would be a problem in the Millennial Kingdom?

Jesus' creation of *wine*. The second event that needs to be considered is found in the narrative of Jesus' first miracle at Cana of Galilee. Here, Jesus made water into *wine*, which a great many modern-day preachers, Bible teachers, and laymen use to legitimize moderate drinking for Christians today, teaching that "if Jesus made it and drank it, it certainly is alright for us."

There is no question of the importance of how this passage is interpreted. Peter Lumpkins, who wrote an exhaustive book on wine in the Bible, says that if Jesus made and drank wine in John 2, then that is the key to the Bible permitting moderate drinking:

> Indisputably the nail most often driven to morally fasten the recreational consumption of intoxicating beverages into a solid ethical structure originates in the New Testament. The Founder of Christianity Himself, the Second Person of the Blessed Trinity, God in human flesh-Jesus Christ-becomes the moderationist model. His practice, they say, unmistakably included consuming intoxicating beverages

himself, and that, in the text before us, actually creating intoxicating beverages for others to consume.[90]

We must answer the question here: was the "wine" that Jesus created really grape juice?

The fact that all Scripture has as a primary subject, the person of Jesus Christ (perfect God, sinless man) will help us to decide the meaning of "wine" in this context. The whole truth about Jesus' first miracle, in John 2, will clarify the issue.

First, Jesus knew the Old Testament Scriptures. He astounded the learned Jews in the temple at the age of twelve. He certainly knew what God said about the effects of alcohol:

Wine is a mocker, strong drink is raging; and whosoever is deceived is not wise ... (Prov. 20:1).

Who hath woe? who hath sorrow? who hath contentions? who hath babbling? who hath wounds without cause? who hath red-ness of eyes? They that tarry long at the wine;... (Prov. 23:29).

Can we imagine that Jesus wanted to produce this effect at the marriage feast? He also would have known specifically the instruction of Habakkuk 2:15:

Woe unto him that giveth his neighbour drink, that puttest thy bottle to him, and makes him drunken also, that thou mayest look on their nakedness!

Obviously, the prophet here is talking about the alcoholic beverage made from grape juice. If *wine* in the Bible always refers to an alcoholic beverage, then Jesus made a drink which certainly contributed to drunkenness. In this case, John says he did this after they had *"well* drunk!" According to God's condemnation in the Old Testament, He would have been clearly at fault for such an act.

There is an equivalent warning about causing people to stumble in Romans 14:21: "It is good neither to eat flesh, nor to drink wine, nor any thing whereby thy brother stumbleth, or is offended, or is made weak."

In the story of the miracle at Cana, the master of the feast says, "Every man at the beginning doth set forth good wine; and when men have well drunk, then that which is worse" (John 2:10). If a person drinks even diluted wine until he has "well drunk," more alcohol will add to the content in his blood and he will be on his way to being "more" drunken.

We have only two possibilities in understanding "wine" in this passage:
1. If they were already drinking unfermented grape juice and He created fresh grape juice, He would have shown His Divine power in creating instantly a natural drink and they could have still tasted grape juice that was better than what they had had!
2. But if they were already drinking alcoholic wine and they were "well drunk" (John says so), and Jesus made more for them, then He created a man-made corruption of a natural drink that made them drunker and incapable of knowing that the created drink was better than what they had already had.

The knowledge of His Holy person and calling make it certain that Jesus would never have created a substance that is systematically condemned in the Old Testament. We must never forget the reason for all of Jesus' miracles-to demonstrate His divine power and glory. In fact, the inspired comment on this miracle is found at the end of the story, John 2:11: This beginning of miracles did

Jesus in Cana, of Galilee, and manifested forth his glory; and his disciples believed on him.

In this chapter we began with God's statement "For the word of the LORD is right; and all his works are done in truth" (Ps. 33:4). God's truth has been given us and we have the responsibility to interpret or understand it correctly. This means to compare Scripture with Scripture, for God often interprets it for us. It also means to respect all of its contexts, grammatical, historical, theological, and Christological. When we do this, we can answer with assurance the question, "Is there grape juice in the Bible?" The answer is an unequivocal "yes" and following chapters will only confirm it.

At the opening of this chapter I spoke of a conversation that I had with a hermeneutics professor who would always answer an emphatic "no" to the possibility that grape juice existed in the Bible. At the end of our time together, after he had rejected all the reasons for affirming "yes," he said, "If you can send me just one proof from an ancient source that I can accept, I will change my mind." After arriving home, I did a study on one Hebrew word, *tirosh*, from the Old Testament and that word is always translated *wine* in the English Bible.[91] I pointed out that reliable French and Italian Bibles translated *tirosh* by a word meaning "must" or freshly squeezed grape juice. The Bible is the oldest and most dependable ancient source available and the Hebrew word *tirosh,* when properly respecting the context and other translations can only be properly translated as "fresh grape juice." I sent this proof to him. Unfortunately, he did not accept it.

X. WRONGLY INTERPRETING "WINE"-A POPULAR ERROR: THE "DILUTED WINE" THEORY

There is a very popular and widespread error in our time, the "Diluted Wine" theory. Those who hold to this theory interpret "wine" in the Bible to be a diluted alcoholic beverage in every passage where God seems to bless "wine" but to be undiluted when God condemns the use thereof. They explain at great length that in Bible times the wine was not nearly as intoxicating as that of today even when it was full strength. Furthermore, according to them, drinking it at that time without diluting it was a social error. Probably, the most widely read author of this theory is Norman Geisler in *A Christian Perspective on Wine Drinking* (in Bibliotheca Sacra, Vol. 139, 1982). Here is a summary of his position:

> The Bible does not teach that New Testament communion wine was unfermented. All wine was fermented wine.
>
> The Bible does not teach that "new wine" was unfermented. Hosea 4:11 says that both "old wine" and "new wine" take away understanding.
>
> It is false to say that Jesus made unfermented wine (compare John 2:9–10 with Mark 2:22 and Eph. 5:18).

> It is incorrect to say that the New Testament teaches that first-century Christians were not to use wine at any time.
>
> It is a myth to say that total abstinence was a New Testament condition for church membership.[92]

His whole argument is based on the presupposition that *wine* is always alcoholic, and he ignores both historical, etymological,[93] and biblical evidence against his position. We will examine several arguments against this interpretation.

1. Historical evidence against "The Diluted Wine Theory."

Much of the "proof" for this theory is an interpretation of historical references that ignores the fact that grape juice syrup was also served by adding water to it. This theory assumes that every time ancient writers talk of adding water they are talking about alcohol. Based on his work, New Testament scholar Robert Stein really exaggerates the theory by saying that wine in the New Testament was essentially purified water: He gives as proof the following statements:

- Wine in Homer's day was twenty parts water to one-part wine.
- Pliny referred to wine as eight parts water to one-part wine.
- Aristophanes: three parts water to two parts wine.
- Euenos: three parts water to one-part wine.
- Hesiod: three parts water to one-part wine.
- Alexis: four parts water to one-part wine.
- Diocles and Anacreon: two parts water to one-part wine.
- Ion: three parts water to one-part wine.
- Strong wine was typically considered to be one-part water to one-part wine.[94]

A great many modern authors take up this refrain with varying statistics and emphasis, but it does not prove this theory.

It is very true that the ancient peoples around the Mediterranean Sea diluted the product of the vine, both alcoholic wine and grape juice. An example of a modern usage of grape juice syrup is given on page 24. There we describe the European use of concentrated grape syrup to which water is added to produce a delicious grape drink. This process goes back as far in history as do vineyards and grape juice. The story of Abigail previously presented also shows the practice of adding water to grape syrup. Many of the historical references given in Stein's list to support the "Diluted Wine theory" could very well have referred to concentrated grape syrup with water. There is absolutely no proof that God blessed diluted wine and condemned undiluted wine.

2. Cultural evidence against "The Diluted Wine Theory."

The assumption that "diluted wine" is always a weak alcoholic drink is untenable in the light of the knowledge of the Old Testament culture. Throughout the biblical presentation of Israel and the Promised Land, there is the description of a special people living in a special land, with conditions that were to be totally different from those of the people around them. God prepared and called out this special people to have a special relationship with Him. In Leviticus 20:26, God says, "And ye shall be holy unto me: for I the LORD am holy, and have severed you from other people, that ye should be mine." He played a large part in determining certain aspects of their culture. They were to love Him and follow His words in obedience while He promised certain blessings to them if they followed Him.

First, God promised a new land to His people when He took them out of slavery in Egypt. He provided this land, according to His promise.

Second, God promised protection of His people, as evidenced by David's statement in Psalms 121:7-8:

> The LORD shall preserve thee from all evil: he shall preserve thy soul. The LORD shall preserve thy going out and thy coming in from this time forth, and even for evermore.

Finally, God promised to provide for the physical needs of His people. Running through the Old Testament, God talked of His provision in terms of natural and healthy products. Two examples of this are the promises to Jacob and to Judah. To Jacob He said, "Therefore God give thee of the dew of heaven, and the fatness of the earth, and plenty of corn and wine" (Gen. 27:28). He told Judah (in Jacob's death-bed blessing to his children) that his inheritance would have both vines and grape juice ("the blood of the grape") in Genesis 49:11.

In all, in the Old Testament, God mentioned bread 255 times, oil 176, fruit or fruit trees 126, corn 86, flour 56, wheat 40, and grapes 30 times. The English word "wine" is found 212 times in the Old Testament and is a translation of seven different Hebrew words. Thirty-one times we find "corn and wine" in a list of several other products mentioned. Twenty-eight times the Hebrew word *tirosh* is used in those lists, which always means fresh grape juice (see page 94).

The God of the Jews promised His people a land which would provide grapes and grape juice. He then provided them with these products and protected them in their land while they enjoyed these products. From all this, we can conclude that what God promised and provided was *not* an alcoholic drink!

3. Scientific and Biblical Evidence against "The Diluted Wine Theory"

One very popular tenet of the "The Diluted Wine Theory" is that diluted alcoholic wine was needed to purify water during Bible times. This idea is expressed in many articles on the world-wide web, and it is often used by Christian writers who have not considered its problems. Garrett Peck, author of *The Prohibition Hangover* (and a freelance writer for the alcoholic beverage industry) says,

> The ancients didn't understand microbes and gas-tro-intestinal disease, but they knew that drinking water led to sickness and sometimes death. The water supply was often contaminated, particularly around settlements that had no sanitation, or even in short supply during droughts. So they drank wine but diluted it with water, both to quench the thirst and to dilute the effects of such strong drink. This kept them healthy. In fact, the phrase "strong drink" in the Bible may refer to undiluted wine.[95]

Even though Peck is not a believer in God's inspired Word and cannot be expected to clearly understand it, that which he espouses so learnedly is repeated by a great many Christian writers, who promote the idea of Christians drinking moderately.

The point that, supposedly, people in Bible times did not have safe drinking water and therefore required alcohol to make it safe is an important point for those who teach that grape juice is never spoken of in the Bible. This supposition is wrong on two counts.

First, it is very clear that there *was* safe drinking water in Bible times and that God made rules for keeping it safe. To show the latter, we will simply remark that God gave very explicit rules for keeping His people well, even to tell them how to keep their camping area clean: "Thou shalt have a place also without the camp, whither thou shalt go forth abroad: and thou shalt have a paddle upon thy weapon; and it shall be, when thou wilt ease thyself abroad, thou shalt dig therewith, and shalt turn back and cover that which cometh from thee" (Deut. 23:12–13).

That water was available can also be easily shown from Scripture. The Bible says, for instance, in Genesis 16:7: "And the angel of the LORD found her by a fountain of water in the wilderness." This was obviously water to drink. Later Abraham gave Hagar a bottle of water and sent her away with her child (Gen. 21:14). Then Rebekah gave Abraham's servant water to drink out of a well (Gen. 24:19). The Bible is full of such references. In fact, Proverbs 5:15 speaks clearly about safe water: "Drink waters out of thine own cistern and running waters out of thine own well." R. A. Baker says, concerning the availability of good water:

> I have read a good many documents of first and second century writers. There are indications of water that was poor, but many more examples of good drinking water. Well water was common, the collection of rain water for drinking was common-the Bible has numerous examples of people drinking water. In the midst of [his] lengthy discourse on wine Pliny admits,... "more labour is spent [on wine]-as if nature had not given us the most healthy of beverages to drink, water, which all other animals make use of ..." [96]

Secondly, to make drinking water safe by adding fermented grape juice is not a process that is used today and there is no proof that it was either possible or in use in Bible times. I have no written proof of this, but there is no historical evidence that families needed to purify drinking water in such a fashion. Boiling water for drinking would have been much easier than preparing enough wine to purify it. As missionaries in Africa, we boiled our water. I called an expert on the purification of water in third world countries to ask her about the possibility of purifying water by mixing in some weak wine. She just laughed at the suggestion. I asked her what percentage of alcohol would have to be added to make unsafe water safe. She said 100% proof! Practically, it would be a very laborious process for each family to have such "purified" water.

R. A. Baker, who does not believe in the "two-wine" understanding of the Bible still did a study on the "diluted wine by water for safety" argument which very often is cited as proof that all "wine" in the Bible is alcoholic:

> The evidence found in most articles to support the idea that the ancient world used wine to make water safe to drink are seriously flawed. Wine was indeed diluted with water, but the purpose was not to make the water safe. People in the ancient world drank water consistently...

This study goes on to quote a survivalist named Miles Stair:

> I can find no official source for sterilizing water with wine-no reference at all that would even hint at the efficacy of such a combination.[97]

It would be well to consider some of the implications of the theory that diluted wine mixed with water made it safe for drinking by God's people.

One such implication concerns the Israelites during their wilderness wanderings. It is unlikely that there could be found enough grapes to process to make enough wine to purify water for the whole congregation for a period of forty years.

Another implication concerns Israel in the Promised Land at the time of David's numbering of the people. When David ordered Joab to number Israel (2 Sam. 24:10) he found 1,250,000 men of war. We can conservatively estimate the population of Israel with women and children during that time to be at least four million. The human body needs approximately 32 oz. of water per day. Even at a 50% mixture of 4% alcohol and water it is impossible that unsafe water would become safe.[77] If we assume that it would then be safe anyway, this would necessitate 10 to 15 oz. of wine per day for four million people: at just 10 oz. per day, this makes twenty million US quarts of wine made and consumed per day! This one calculation makes this theory absolutely untenable.

Moreover, we could ask some very disturbing questions of those who affirm that people in Bible times mixed fermented wine with unsafe water to make it safe. For instance, "Would it have been healthy for pregnant mothers to drink that much alcohol?" and "How about children?"

And what about, "Why were the Nazirites and the Rechabites denied the protection of mixing wine with their water?" God told them they could not drink of the fruit of the vine!

Whether intoxicating wine was diluted in Bible times or not has no bearing on the question of whether or not grape juice existed at that time and was available. We know that concentrated grape juice was mixed with water from the story of Abigail and the feast she brought David and his eighty men (see page 24). We also know that some people got drunk on biblical "wine," proving that their wine could have sufficient alcohol for drunkenness.

4. Hermeneutical Evidence against "The Diluted Wine Theory."

We have already shown that the word *wine* in the Bible is a generic word which is used to refer to several different Hebrew words meaning grape juice or alcoholic wine. We have presented arguments showing that the Diluted Wine theory is a wrong interpretation of biblical "wine." Now we want to consider the phrase "wine and strong drink" as used in Scripture.

A proper interpretation of this phrase will reveal the "diluted wine theory" as fallacy. The popular teaching is that "wine" in the Bible is usually diluted and that "strong drink" then would indicate undiluted wine. In the English Bible, the Hebrew word for this drink, is *shaycawr*, and has been translated by the two words "strong drink."

> As to the words "strong drink" in our common version, it may here be well to remark, that there are not two words in the original, but only the one word, "Shecar" or "Shaycaw." One learned author says, that the primitive idea of meaning of the word is: "sweetness," and this "sweet drink," as he renders it, was produced from the palm tree.[98]

This term is wrongly understood by some modern writers to refer to strong alcoholic content. In fact, some translate it "intoxicating drink." This incorrect translation is a result of failure to apply Bible etymology. Just as the word "wine" in the Bible is generic, so also is "strong drink." It can refer to a grain drink or a palm drink and either could be fermented or not.

Shaycawr, or "strong drink" in the Authorized Version, is mentioned twenty times in the Old Testament. Except for one, every verse that contains it speaks also of *wine*, usually as a synonym. Sometimes its use is condemned and sometimes it is condoned. This would prove that in each case they are both either alcoholic or both non-alcoholic. The first case is clearly shown through many references. For instance, Isaiah spoke of both wine and strong drink in Isaiah. 28:7:

> But they also have erred through wine, and
> through strong drink are out of the way; the priest
> and the prophet have erred through strong drink,
> they are swallowed up of wine, they are out of the
> way through strong drink; they err in vision, they
> stumble in judgment.

Both of these terms in this verse are synonyms in the sense that their effects are harmful.

There are also many references which refer to both of these drinks as being beneficial and non-alcoholic. God told His people to pour this drink (Shaycawr) out before Him as a drink offering in Numbers 28:7, and we know there was to be no leaven in drink offerings. In Deuteronomy 14:26, it is included in the list of acceptable things they could bring before Him to eat or drink as an act of worship:

> And thou shalt bestow that money for whatsoever
> thy soul lusteth after, for oxen, or for sheep, or for
> wine, or for strong drink, or for whatsoever thy soul
> desireth: and thou shalt eat there before the LORD
> thy God, and thou shalt rejoice, thou, and thine
> household.

This makes no sense if Shaycawr referred to a "strong" alcoholic beverage as most Christian writers propose. Remember, the writers who promote the "one-wine" theory believe that God only blessed wine diluted with water and that Shaycawr, or "strong drink," represented undiluted wine. This is not true according to the meaning of Shaycawr, and it is not true according to Bible usage. God commanded His people to drink both Shaycawr and "wine" before His altar! We must understand that "strong drink" in the Old Testament referred to a sweet drink which was not usually fermented but could be. It was not a product of the vine. Many pastors who have accepted the current "diluted wine" teaching are simply unaware that Shaycawr is mentioned with wine in Scripture as an acceptable offering to God.

The mixture of gleanings from ancient writings and the modern rationale which is found in the Diluted Wine theory solves no problem in the understanding of "wine" in the Bible. The Bible is the inerrant, inspired Revelation of the Holy God who clearly condemns intoxicating wine. The analysis of the Jewish culture and the historical situation of God's people finds no place for the widespread use of alcoholic beverages, no matter how diluted. Alcohol does not fit with the other basic, natural, healthy products that God provided for His people. Diluting a glass of intoxicating wine still leaves a percentage of alcohol in the drink and alcohol is a poison for the human system.

In our discussion of the sacrifices, we talked about the necessity of making sure there was no leaven present in those sacrifices. When we talk about the presence or absence of leaven or yeast in the drink offerings it matters little whether or not the alcohol was diluted. Leaven was always present in diluted alcohol; therefore, the sacrifice would not be acceptable, and the diluted wine theory is once again proved erroneous.

XI. TODAY-A GROWING PROBLEM WITH ALCOHOL

E ven those who espouse the use of alcohol in moderation must agree that alcohol is an enormous problem in our modern culture. The list of comments about its dangers given previously on page xxii shows the seriousness of this social ill in our time. Even more frightening than the actual dangers that the consumption of alcohol creates in society is the fact that society in America has rapidly and fundamentally changed its attitude towards this consumption. Startling differences can be seen between the early 1900s, 1950–1980, and the early 2000s. Even greater changes can be foreseen as the problem worsens.

1. Societal and Christian attitudes toward alcoholic consumption in the early 1900s.

During the 100 years before 1900, a fierce battle waged between those engaged in either the sale or consumption of alcoholic beverages (including some church leaders) and the citizens, churches, and Christian organizations who were against it. The issue was hotly debated, especially among those in religious circles. We have seen in a preceding chapter that the *wets* (proponents of alcoholic consumption) were quite categorical in their attacks on the *dries* (proponents of temperance).

The *"dries"* were militantly against the consumption of alcohol. They spoke vehemently against the "modern" biblical interpretation of their time which trumpeted that *wine* in the Bible was always alcoholic. They wrote and spoke at length on the subject.

Three quotations from Eliphalet Nott in 1847 will serve to illustrate their teachings:

> That the fruit of the vine, in the form of grape juice as expressed from the cluster, has been from remote antiquity and still is used as a beverage, is abundantly in proof. [99]

Concerning God's blessing and condemning the same substance, Nott says,

> Can the same thing in the same state be good and bad, a symbol of wrath, a symbol of mercy, a thing to be sought after, a thing to be avoided? Certainly not.[100]

Then he asks a question and gives the answer,

> And is the Bible then inconsistent with itself? No it is not, and this seeming inconsistency will vanish, and the Bible will be not only, but will appear to be in harmony with itself, in harmony with history, with science, and with the providence of God...[101]

A popular evangelist, writing on the subject of wine in 1980, characterized the earlier era by saying,

> Many books were written during that period, some of which were by reputable Hebrew and Greek scholars who set forth solid evidence showing that the major words that were translated "wine" in Scripture (Hebrew *yayin*, Greek *oinos*) could mean either fermented or unfermented grape juice.[102]

Peter Lumpkins quoted John J. Owens about the drinking practices of Jesus, saying: "as wine was a common beverage in that
land of vineyards, in its unfermented state, our Lord most likely
drank it. But that he did so in its intoxicating forms or that he
indulged to excess in its use in any form, was a false and malicious
libel upon his character."[103]

Most evangelical churches responded to the teaching of that
era. In 1896 the Southern Baptists passed this resolution:

> Furthermore, we announce it as the sense of this
> body that no person should be retained in the fel-
> lowship of a Baptist church who engages in the
> manufacture or sale of alcoholic liquors, or who
> rents his property to be used for distilleries,.. Nor
> do we believe that any church should retain in its
> fellowship any member who drinks intoxicating
> liquors as a beverage...[104]

A large part of society was arrayed alongside preachers against the use of alcohol at that time. Interest was very high and evangelist Billy Sunday along with others who spoke to the subject drew very large crowds. The

DURING THE PROHIBITION ERA (1919-1933):
- Crime decreased 54%
- The death rate due to liquor decreased 43%
- 97 of the 98 Keeley Alcoholics Clinics closed for lack of patients.
- Insanity decreased 66%

result was that laws on
prohibition were passed, first in several individual states and then
nationally in 1919, and consumption dramatically decreased.[105]
There were also other beneficial results of Prohibition, crime

decreased 54% the death rate due to liquor decreased 43%, 97 of the 98 Keeley Alcoholics Clinics closed for lack of patients, insanity decreased 66%, and all 60 Neil Cure Clinics closed for lack of patients afflicted with alcoholism. An article in the Christian Post, "Prohibition and the Legalization of Drugs," speaks to this issue:

> Contrary to popular opinion, Prohibition was quite successful. It didn't eradicate drinking, but it did significantly reduce consumption rates and thereby improve the public health. In his book "The Devaluing of America," William Bennett, former director of the Office of National Drug Control Policy under President George H.W. Bush, said: "One of the clear lessons of Prohibition is that when we had laws against alcohol there was less consumption, less alcohol-related disease, fewer drunken brawls, and a lot less drunkenness. Contrary to myth, there is no evidence that Prohibition caused any big increases in crime.[106]

To recap, the early 1900s was a time when:

- the evil of drinking was well known in society;
- liberal church leaders endorsed it; evangelicals fought it, preached and taught extensively and successfully against it.

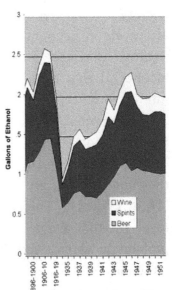

2. Societal and Christian attitudes toward alcoholic consumption from 1950 to 1980.

By 1950, Prohibition was a thing of the past: criticized, repealed and all but forgotten. Of course, we can notice by the graph below that this brought in a new day. Society was once more free-free to buy and consume alcohol, though there were still a few locations where prohibition was in force. One could easily purchase alcoholic beverages even in grocery stores. Massive television advertisement encouraging use of alcohol was just beginning, but its effect was dramatic. There was a surge in drinking, in alcohol abuse, in youth drinking, and in social acceptance of alcohol. In an article in *Times Magazine* (Nov. 5, 1979), the Dean of students at Chicago's Loyola University was quoted as saying, "The single greatest drug abuse on this or any campus is undoubtedly alcohol."[107] The same article goes on to say:

> Some sample results [of a poll] at 34 New England four-year colleges show that more than 95% of the undergraduates report at least occasional drinking, compared with 59% who smoke marijuana, 11% who snort cocaine and 10% who pop tranquilizers.

> Twenty percent of the men and 10% of the women say getting drunk "was important" to them.

> The category of "heavy drinkers"-those who regularly consume more than a six-pack of beer or five shots of liquor at a sitting-now includes 29% of undergraduate men and 11% of the women.

This terrible condition was only beginning to manifest itself in 1950, and the problem was full-blown by 1980.

There are two facts that came to light during this time: the fact that consumption of alcohol was beginning to be accepted by a significant portion of American society and the frightening fact that the evangelical churches in America had abandoned their role of warning society against this public menace.

A quote from a popular evangelist's book written in 1980 will illustrate the first fact. Quoted earlier in this chapter, he describes how a marriage that started so well went so drastically downhill due to alcohol abuse that the wife was desperate. This anecdote speaks of one particular case but is found to be true of hundreds of thousands of cases throughout society.

> First, they had enjoyed a few beers together. "Nobody gets drunk on beer," he had said. Before long, beer present for every evening... it became the drink to serve when friends dropped in.
>
> When he had begun to climb in the company, there was entertaining to be done. "Social drinking."
>
> His drinking had increased. When he wanted to stop drinking, he couldn't. She was sick of his drinking, of his lies, of his broken promises.[108]

The second fact, that the evangelical churches in America had abandoned their role of warning society, is harder to document since the "absence" of something is always hard to prove. It is clear, however, that evangelical leaders were not speaking out or writing on the subject. In 1950, as far as I can discover, there was not one single book on the market in America which proved that grape juice was in the Bible and that God did not condone moderate drinking. The only book dealing with the subject, (out of print for a long time and since republished), was Rev. William Patton's book, *Bible Wines or the Laws of Fermentation and Wines of the Ancients*. Robert Teachout's book, *Wine The Biblical Imperative: Total Abstinence*, based on his doctoral thesis, was published in 1983.

And yet, in 1950, evangelical churches were still living in the shadow of all the teaching and preaching of the proceeding era, and they almost universally lived and promoted abstinence. Most evangelical churches included in their church covenants a statement on this. Though there was little teaching on the central issue of the proper interpretation of the Bible words for grape juice and wine, there was an emphasis on purity and a consensus that alcohol and its effects were bad, and a Christian should not partake. This consensus was not at all shared by the liberal denominations. It was a blessing that abstinence was still the norm among evangelical churches, and this was definitely the result of the battle for abstinence during and preceding the Prohibition eras. The tragic side of this "blessed fact" of temperance being in church statements of faith was that a standard of living was promoted and even required, but there was no teaching to align it with the Bible. Maintaining a standard of abstinence without attaching it to biblical teaching led to either legalism or abandonment of the standard.

To recap, 1950 to 1980 was a time when:
- the evil of drinking was well known in society and was increasing dramatically among the youth;
- liberal church leaders endorsed it;
- some evangelical leaders began promoting moderate consumption;
- most evangelical churches still practiced abstinence;
- teaching that grape juice is in the Bible and that God condemned alcoholic beverages was almost unknown.

3. Societal and Christian attitudes toward alcoholic consumption in the early 2000s.

An enormous change took place in evangelical churches by the year 2000. This change could be likened to a tsunami. Jaeggli says, (citing a survey of nine evangelical liberal-arts colleges and seven seminaries): "In 1951, 98% of students in these institutions agreed that it was always wrong to drink Alcohol, but that percentage dropped to only 17% by 1982."[109]

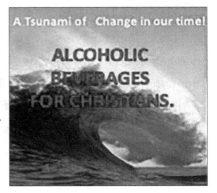

Undoubtedly, today the percentage would be even lower, because church leaders and biblical scholars no longer warn about the dangers of alcohol. They began to write and to teach about the wrongness of abstinence and the biblical reasons for moderate drinking. Even those who still espoused abstinence defended the one-wine theory of Bible interpretation and the resulting teaching that Jesus made and drank an alcoholic beverage. This teaching came at a time when society was becoming completely complacent about the sale and consumption of alcohol. While law enforcement agencies fought the effects, drinking itself was universally accepted in society as a whole and more and more among Christians. How much society changed in just fifty years is amazing!

There are three specific changes that brought about the overall transformation: the bombardment of advertising encouraging alcohol consumption, increased consumption of alcohol among the youth, and a continued shift in the attitude of most evangelical churches toward alcoholic beverages-the abandonment of abstinence. These changes will be considered at length in the following pages.

4. Bombardment of advertising encouraging alcohol consumption.

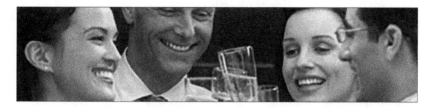

By the year 2000, most Americans had color television and spent many hours watching it. This made the constant stream of advertising of alcoholic products not only present in every home but made these products seem very innocuous, interesting, and enticing. Although society was now officially aware of the dangers of tobacco, there were no warnings attached to alcoholic products, even though numerous studies showed the increased danger of alcohol consumption. It was always presented as an important and necessary part of social activities and a healthy and satisfying way to find happiness. Advertisers routinely promoted health, fun, and sex with their advertisements which targeted youth.

This adver-tising blitz has advanced since 2000. Advertising companies are now searching for ways to invade the iPhones of the

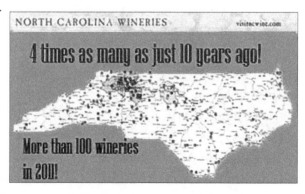

NORTH CAROLINA WINERIES   visitncwine.com

4 times as many as just 10 years ago!

More than 100 wineries in 2011!

youth with advertisements of alcoholic beverages! This advertising has resulted in a dramatic increase in sales of all alcoholic bever-ages, but it has perhaps caused the greatest increase in the sale of wine. One winery in North Carolina boasts "80 years ago we bottled MOONSHINE. Now we bottle sunshine!" The graphic on the increase of wineries in NC will show this increase.

5. Increased consumption of alcohol among the youth.

In the introduction we quoted two shocking statistics:
- ✓ One quarter of American teenagers are into "binge drinking."
- ✓ By the age of sixteen most kids will have seen 75,000 ads for alcohol. Young people view 20,000 commercials each year, and nearly 2,000 are for beer and wine.

Does this advertising succeed? Very definitely-if it did not, the producers would not pay the enormous cost for advertising their products. We do not have to wonder at its success; recent studies have documented it:

> A study found that, among a group of 2,250 middle-school students in Los Angeles, those who viewed more television programs containing alcohol commercials while in the seventh grade were more likely in the eighth grade to drink beer, wine/liquor, or to drink three or more drinks on at least one occasion during the month prior to the follow-up survey.

> Researchers followed 3,111 students in S. Dakota from seventh to ninth grade, and found that exposure to in-store beer displays in grade 7 predicted onset of drinking by grade 9, and exposure to magazine advertising for alcohol at sports or music events predicted frequency of drinking in grade 9.[110]

When one thinks of the message of these commercials-fun and sex without limit-one can understand the appeal. The scary part of this is that the drinking problem is getting worse. With the demise of the church as a restraining factor there is nothing to inhibit the producers or the consumers. Liberal society is trying to take away legal restraints and allow even younger youths to consume Alcohol. As proof of this, you can google "Amethyst Initiative." I quote here from their web page:

> Launched in July 2008, the Amethyst Initiative is made up of chancellors and presidents of universities and colleges across the United States. These higher education leaders have signed their names to a public statement that the problem of irresponsible drinking by young people continues despite the minimum legal drinking age of 21, and there is a culture of dangerous binge drinking on many campuses.
>
> The Amethyst Initiative supports informed and unimpeded debate on the 21-year-old drinking age...[111]

In their statement, they declare that "it's time to rethink the drinking age [because] twenty-one is not working."[112] They want to lower it to 18.

Even though there are still laws against underage drinking, consider this:

> Not only did underage drinkers consume 11 percent of all alcoholic beverages purchased in the United States in 2002, but also the vast majority of the alcohol purchased for underage consumption was consumed in binge and heavy drinking.[113]

6. A continued shift in the attitude of most evangelical churches toward alcoholic beverages and toward the abandonment of abstinence.

It was mentioned in the introduction that Bible colleges are changing their teaching on the consumption of alcohol. By 1950 the teaching about the presence of grape juice in the Bible and God's condemnation of all alcoholic beverages had all but disappeared, though abstinence was still being taught and was found in most evangelical church constitutions. By the early 2000s, there were voices being raised to actively promote moderate drinking in evangelical circles and to aggressively attack those who would continue to teach abstinence. Even those who do still stand for abstinence do not teach the position that not all "wine" in the Bible is alcoholic.

Since it would be a lengthy process to quote from so many leaders of the different denominations, the demonstration of the dramatic turn towards consumption of alcohol will be limited to the Southern Baptist Convention. This is because the SBC held to a position on abstinence longer than most other groups and because it is the largest group. Peter Lumpkins, a Southern Baptist minister and writer, has done much research on the recent change in the position of the SBC. He says concerning the historical position of the SBC,

> beginning in 1886 up until 2006, no fewer than 40 resolutions have been passed by Southern Baptists (Richard Land, 2008). All of these presumably presented the same message: total abstinence from alcoholic beverages for pleasurable purposes.[114]

The following quotes about the present message of many SBC leaders are from Lupkin's book, *Alcohol Today: Abstinence in an Age of Indulgence*:

> The Christian Church (especially the Protestant side) that was virtually unanimous in support of the "old, failed Prohibition" policies will go on record quickly these days, if asked, that imbibing alcoholic beverages is not as bad as it used to be (p. 19).

> One professor from a Southern Baptist seminary had this to say, "Are alcoholic beverages a good thing? Sure. Within moderate amounts, of course. In fact, don't ever let anyone tell you any differently. If they do, they are closet Roman Catholics who are imposing pharisaical legalism on you. They do not hold to Scripture" (p. 20).

> "The idea that to drink a glass of wine, or any other alcoholic beverage, is a sin against God is so foreign to the teaching of the inspired, inerrant Word of God that for anyone to say to a Christian who has no conviction about drinking alcoholic beverages, 'You are sinning against God when you drink a glass of wine' is a sin itself" (p. 33, quoting president of Baptist General Convention of Oklahoma).

> The approaching crisis for Southern Baptists concerns behavior-a cataclysmal moral shift away from the biblical holiness expressed in biblical Lordship, toward the relativistic postmodern norms of American pop culture, including its hedonistic obsession with fulfilling desires (p. 34, 35).[115]

Since the Southern Baptist Convention is the largest Baptist denomination in the world, the changes in their official position are significant and reveal a trend that is probably even more advanced in all the rest of evangelical churches, though some still hold to abstinence.

To recap, societal and Christian attitudes toward alcoholic consumption by the early 2000s has evolved dramatically and that in just 50 years. It has been a time when:

- the evil of drinking alcohol has become accepted as normal in society and the youth lead the way in "pushing the envelope";
- liberal church leaders continue to endorse freedom to drink alcoholic beverages;
- many evangelical leaders promote moderate consumption of alcohol;
- other evangelicals neither fight it nor preach and teach against it;
- few evangelical churches practice abstinence aggressively;
- the teaching that grape juice is in the Bible is attacked by all but a very few.

In order to fully understand God's teaching on this subject, we must examine more closely what the Bible says about moderate drinking.

XII. MODERATE CONSUMPTION OF ALCOHOL

In chapter II it was mentioned that most of the Radio dramatizations of Pacific Garden Mission during the 1950s were stories of professional men with families who started out with light (or moderate) social drinking and then went on to become down-and-out bums on skid row where they found the Savior and gave up their alcohol. In Chapter XII, I will cite a story of a man who started with moderate drinking and went on to alcoholic dependence and a failing marriage. The fact is that very few people start drinking moderately with the goal of arriving at alcohol abuse, but that is often what happens.

Today there are a great many proponents of moderate drinking for health and other reasons, and many of its proponents are Christian writers and leaders.

Before we go further, it would be wise to ask the question, "Why would one want to begin drinking moderately, or as Eliphalet Nott puts it in his 'Lectures on Temperance'?"

> What is the cause of moderate or temperate drinking? Is it the force of natural appetite? Rarely. Nine-tenths, if not nineety-nine hundredths, of those who use alcoholic stimulants, do it in the first instance, and often for a long time, *not from appetite, but from deference to custom or fashion.* Usage has associated intoxicating drinks with good fellowship-with offices of hospitality and friendship.[116]

Here we will discuss four elements of the question: "Should Christians start drinking alcohol moderately?" We will find that moderate drinking is not a healthy addition to a person's diet, that moderate drinking is dangerous, that moderate drinking can lead to serious consumption of alcoholic beverages, and that there are proponents of moderate drinking among Christian leaders in spite of the dangers.

1. Moderate Drinking Does Not Have Health Benefits.

Here, we are questioning a very popular scientific "fact," that drinking wine *does* have health benefits, a "fact" that is repeated often on the internet, in blogs, and other literature. We disagree and make the following statement on good authority and note that this is not a personal conclusion:

> An Addiction Specialist and Senior Scientist at the Centre for Addiction and Mental Health at the University of Toronto states that "the health benefits of alcohol use are generally overstated and are virtually nonexistent for young people. Even small amounts of alcohol increase the risk of injury and boost the chances of developing about sixty diseases.[117]

The key here is that even *if* there were health benefits, we would say, "Watch out for the side effects. Watch out for the effects of the poison you would put in your body and its subsequent consequences."

But there is a simple and very scientific answer to all the promotion of wine as a simple health producer. The benefits are in the grape juice! An article put on the web by CNN Health reports:

> If you don't like wine, the latest studies show you
> can get almost all the same benefits from grape
> juice. The reason [is that] purple grape juice con-
> tains the same powerful disease-fighting antioxi-
> dants, called flavonoids, that are believed to give
> wine many of its heart-friendly benefits...[118]

This report quotes a study published in 1999 in the journal circulation, in which researchers at the University of Wisconsin Medical School in Madison asked fifteen patients to drink a tall glass of grape juice daily.

> After 14 days, blood tests revealed that LDL oxi-
> dation in these patients was significantly reduced.
> And ultrasound images showed changes in the
> artery walls, indicating that their blood was flowing
> more freely.

> Grape juice can also lower the risk of developing
> the blood clots that lead to heart attacks .Wine only
> prevents blood from clotting when it's consumed
> at levels high enough to declare someone legally
> drunk, says University of Wisconsin researcher
> John Folts, PhD. With grape juice, you can drink
> enough to get the benefit without worrying about
> becoming intoxicated.

2. Moderate Drinking Is Dangerous.

There are those in society and especially in law enforcement who are very much aware of the dangers of moderate drinking. This awareness has been in existence for a very long time. A state-ment in a *School Physiology Journal* in 1901 states:

I affirm that a man who abstains totally from the use of alcoholic drinks does not deny himself anything; he gains in the blessing and joy of life. No drunkard was ever saved by the resolution to become a moderate drinker. Salvation consists in avoiding the first glass. The moderate drinker tempts others. It is not the drunkards who lead men astray; they rather have the great merit of deterring others by their example.

Those who lead others into temptation are the moderate drinkers. And so long as this temptation continues there will be no end to intemperance and its results, namely, disease, insanity, and crime. Whoever fails to recognize this fact does not understand the history of the warfare against intemperance.[119]

> The moderate drinker tempts others!

In modern times we can be more technical. Here are some statements by the Mayo Clinic and the AMA:

Alcohol use disorder (which includes a level that's sometimes called alcoholism) is a pattern of alcohol use that involves problems controlling your drinking, being preoccupied with alcohol, continuing to use alcohol even when it causes problems, having to drink more to get the same effect, or having withdrawal symptoms when you rapidly decrease or stop drinking.[120]

Many people begin to drink alcohol during ado-
lescence and young adulthood. Alcohol consumption during this developmental period may have
profound effects on brain structure and function.
Heavy drinking has been shown to affect the neu-
ropsychological performance (e.g., memory func-
tions) of young people and may impair the growth
and integrity of certain brain structures.[121]

When alcohol reaches the brain, it doesn't kill the cells. What
it does is inhibit the communication between dendrites, or branching
connections at the ends of neurons that send and receive information between neurons, in the cerebellum, a part of the brain
involved in motor coordination. This poor communication results
in some of the typical impairments of intoxication.[122]

A new study, (Sept. 13, 2018), says:

This might not be the answer people want to hear,
but there is no safe level for drinking alcohol. Of
course there is lower-risk drinking, but WHO does
not set particular limits, because the evidence
shows that the ideal situation for health is to not
drink at all.[123]

In some ways, the particular danger of drinking alcohol is that
it leads to a lessoning of the control of our conscience and encourages one to go against his inhibitions, which outweighs the dangers to health and the risks of death. As dangerous as are these
two elements of the problem, the fact that one's upbringing, God-
given conscious, and learned aversion to evil can all be quickly
set aside by a glass of alcohol, to be replaced by an urge to do

something which is counter to one's convictions is frightening. To put it in more scientific terms, we cite from *Psychology Today*.

> A subsequent group of researchers found that drinking increases levels of norepinephrine, the neurotransmitter responsible for arousal, which would account for heightened excitement when someone begins drinking. Elevated levels of norepinephrine increase impulsivity, which helps explain why we lose our inhibitions [to] drinking. Drunken brains are primed to seek pleasure without considering the consequences; no wonder so many hook-ups happen after happy hour.[124]

This process begins immediately as alcohol is ingested.

3. Moderate drinking can lead to serious consumption of alcoholic beverages

The Massachusetts report cited in the Appendix goes further to make further pertinent statements:

> In addition to the potential individual consequences of increased alcohol consumption, the public may suffer from the promotion of moderate drinking.

> Although drinking is a personal act and an individual responsibility, it is also behavior shaped by our societies and something for which society as a whole has responsibility." According to the World Health Organization, "measures that influence drinkers in general will also have an impact on heavier drinkers. Promoting increased levels of

moderate drinking may in turn increase overall consumption, even for those who should not do so.[125]

The government defines moderate drinking as "one drink per day for women and two drinks per day for men." This becomes vital if one exceeds permitted levels of alcohol in the blood, since most states now have very severe penalties for driving under the influence. At this point we need to be very clear what moderate drinking is for a Christian.

What is moderate drinking by Bible standards? We are constantly reminded by those who teach the one-wine theory that wine in the Bible had a much lower alcohol content than today's alcoholic beverages.

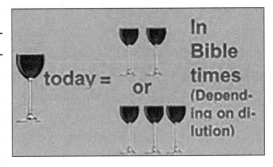

Without going through the necessary mathematical equations, we can say that one glass of wine today has the alcohol equivalent of two or three glasses in Bible times.

First, when we look at the effects of moderate drinking in society today, the dangers are very clear. "One more for the road" is not a wise choice. The news reports are constantly assailing us

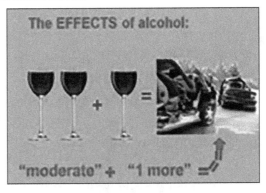

with tragedies that happen suddenly, after the faculties have been impaired by alcohol.

Two Wines: A Proper Understanding of "Wine" in the Bible

Secondly, the influence of moderate social drinking on families is very great. When children are taught by their parents' example that a "celebration" requires alcohol for the adults or that a full meal requires alcohol for the parents, children develop a desire

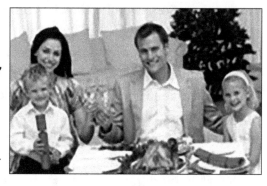

to be able to one day partake in that adult activity. Of course, if they are permitted to taste the alcohol at the table, it becomes just that much worse. They are totally unprotected the first time they are offered alcohol in an unsupervised situation.

4. Proponents of moderate drinking among Christian authors and leaders.

In spite of the well-known dangers of moderate drinking, there are an increasing number of Christians who forcefully defend it. The default view of the church today about the recreational consumption of intoxicating beverages, according to Peter Lumpkins, is **moderation**. He says that the mantra is very clear and memorable for all who defend the thesis that wine in the Bible is always alcoholic. They insist that the Bible condemns the abuse of intoxicating drink, not the use of intoxicating drink.[126]

A blog on moderate drinking sums up the attitude of many:

> Drinking socially-not "getting drunk"-can be an opportunity to demonstrate the Gospel message. Christians who drink with restraint show that they're strong enough in their faith to be controlled

by God and not be slaves to alcohol, food or other worldly desires...

Christian groups across the spectrum, from Catholics to non-denominational congregations, have started new ministries to bring together beer and the Bible, to put "theology on tap." They're meeting in bars, serving booze at Bible study and inserting their message into places where communities are already forming, reaching people where they are rather than forcing them into a church building.[127]

This is a view with growing popularity, and those who try to combat it are often reviled.

Most Christian leaders who espouse moderate drinking for Christians today are using Scripture to defend their thesis. Most of these Christian leaders will also say that a proper drink in Bible times was always greatly diluted. However, one drink today already has the alcoholic content of two or three drinks in Bible times, leading to the conclusion that the Bible cannot support the moderate drinking of today.

This brings us back to the question, "Should Christians start drinking alcohol moderately?" If one chooses to ignore the dangers and teach one's children to do likewise, one will advance in the direction of moderate drinking. If one wants to take seriously the dangers of alcohol and the admonitions of the Lord, one will abstain and teach his children to do likewise.

XIII. THE IMPORTANCE OF ABSTINENCE FOR THE CHRISTIAN

The word "abstinence" has been made a pejorative word in our times, almost a fighting word, between those who are convinced that God approves moderate drinking and those who are convinced of the contrary. Human history, however, shows us a great many instances where abstinence has been required. Field provides this historical data with sources:

> Two thousand years before Christ it was enjoined upon the Egyptian Priesthood. Centuries later, the Institutes of Menu required it of all officiating Brahmins. In the "Pentalogue of Buddha" (BC 560) there ran this precept: "Thou shalt not drink any intoxicating liquor."[128]

Even in our era, for the good of the bodies of competing athletes, alcohol is forbidden.

Beyond the questions concerning the interpretation of God's Word, there is a very important matter of application. Over seventy-five years ago there was a turning away from that interpretation which affirmed the actuality of grape juice in the Bible to that which mandated only alcohol. Some modern writers continue this "belief" and enlarge it to affirm that in Bible times those who pleased God drank "moderately," so Christians may drink moderately today. Yet some of those who feel this way still believe that it is best to abstain altogether.

Many who do believe in moderation say that we must warn people to be moderate, but we must be careful not to speak too much about the dangers of alcoholic beverages so as not to offend anyone. These same Christians would never moderately react if their children were running out into the street. They would never moderately wake their family up if their house was on fire. And yet they will teach their children that they can drink moderately of a product that is deliberately produced to attack the powers of judgment.

It is often considered that "moderate" means only one or two glasses of an alcoholic beverage, but this would mean that a person is always just one glass removed from going beyond moderate. It seems that wisdom itself demands that we not even take the risk of trying to keep it "under control." Consider the authoritative and inspired wisdom of Proverbs 23:31-33: "Look not thou upon the wine when it is red, when it giveth his colour in the cup, when it moveth itself aright. At the last it biteth like a serpent, and stingeth like an adder." Going against this Scriptural warning, whoever practices "moderate drinking" and tries to not go beyond, puts himself unwisely within reach of getting bit by the "serpent-like" wine.

Christians need to speak out concerning the dangers of alcoholic beverages. Scientific articles continue to do so. An article on the web speaks directly to the danger of even a small amount of alcohol:[129]

> The brain is the body's control center... The brain is part of a body system called the Central Nervous System, or CNS ... While all body systems feel the effects of alcohol, the CNS is particularly sensitive.... The first areas affected by small amounts of alcohol are those involved in inhibiting behaviors, which can cause an increase in animation, an increase in talkativeness, and greater sociability....Here are indications that the brain is slowing down:

- · Altered speech
- · Hazy thinking
- · Slowed reaction time
- · Dulled hearing
- · Impaired vision

Author Jim McGuiggan goes on to quote a scientist who discusses drinking and driving: "The drinker is in the worst possible position to make the decision whether he is safe to drive or not... Alcohol is detectable in the brain within a half a minute after being swallowed."[130] In fact, the drinker is in no position to make any moral decisions at all. A Christian should never be in such a position (see 1 Pet. 1:13, 4:7; 5:8; Tit. 2:6).

Those who teach their children to drink moderately leave them totally unprotected when they go out with friends who do not drink moderately.

The same web page quotes Joseph A. Califano Jr., Chairman and President of the National Center on Addiction and Substance Abuse at Columbia University as saying, "A child who reaches age 21 without smoking, abusing alcohol or using drugs is virtually certain never to do so."

Actually, in discussing the dangers of alcohol, we must go even further. Many Christians are aware of the danger of becoming an alcoholic. It has often been said that taking a drink of an alcoholic beverage is like playing Russian roulette because one doesn't know if he will become addicted or not.

But alcohol is very dangerous for even those who are *not* addicted. There is always the danger of alcohol abuse. Many do not know that there is a difference between alcoholic addiction and abuse:

Alcohol **addiction** refers to a psychological dependence on alcohol that involves continued,

> compulsive drinking that does not stop despite adverse consequences...

> Alcohol **abusers** are not necessarily addicted to alcohol. Abusers are typically heavy drinkers of alcohol who continue drinking regardless of the results. Abusers of alcohol may not drink on a consistent basis.[131]

In other words, you do not have to be addicted to alcohol to abuse alcohol. You can be a moderate, occasional alcohol consumer who finds himself with the wrong group and one drink leads to another and it has turned into a "binge" and you have abused alcohol. Consider a high school student who has been taught that drinking in itself is not wrong. Then he finds himself with the wrong friends, has just three drinks, and has a fatal accident on the way home.

The American Psychological Association defines alcohol abuse in this way:

> **Alcohol abuse** is a drinking pattern that results in significant and recurrent adverse consequences. Alcohol abusers may fail to fulfill major school, work, or family obligations. They may have drinking-related legal problems, such as repeated arrests for driving while intoxicated. They may have relationship problems related to their drinking.[132]

Many do not realize that there is the danger of alcohol abuse for *all* who drink moderately. A recent television show on the health channel gave the three top causes of death in the USA: smoking, obesity, and alcohol abuse (not alcoholism). Alcohol abuse leads to disease, accidents, and crimes which stem from any use of alcohol. "Worldwide alcohol use and abuse statistics are staggering. The single highest risk factor for premature death and disability for individuals between 15 and 49 years old across the world is alcohol abuse."[133]

The dramatic difference between smoking, obesity, and alcohol abuse is that those who indulge in obesity and smoking essentially only harm themselves-that is bad enough!-but alcohol abuse is often the direct cause of death and suffering for totally innocent persons.

> Alcoholism, now known as alcohol use disorder, is a condition in which a person has a desire or physical need to consume alcohol, even though it has a negative impact on their life.

> In the past, a person with this condition was referred to as an "alcoholic." However, this is increasingly seen as an unhelpful and negative label. Health professionals now say that a person has an Alcohol Use Disorder (AUD).

> According to the National Institute of Health (NIH), in 2015, 15.1 million American adults (6.2 percent of the population) had an alcohol use problem.

> According to the World Health Organization (WHO), globally, 3.3 million deaths every year result from the harmful use of alcohol.[134]

The extreme danger of alcohol abuse is that it does not take a regular pattern of drinking to be lethal. Just one episode is enough to ruin many lives.

When we look at statistics of drinking by American youth, they are simply terrifying. The National Institute on Alcohol Abuse and Alcoholism gives the following statistics:

> People ages 12 through 20 drink 11 percent of all alcohol consumed in the United States. Although youth drink less often than adults do, when they do drink, they drink more. That is because young people consume more than 90 percent of their alcohol by binge drinking.
>
> By age 15, about 33 percent of teens have had at least one drink.
>
> By age 18, about 60 percent of teens have had at least one drink.

The results of all this drinking are shocking. From 2006 to 2010 the CDC reported an average of 4,368 young people died under the age of 21 and 188,000 people under age 21 visited an emergency room for alcohol-related injuries.[135] Finally, in 2015, 7.7 million young people ages 12–20 reported that they drank alcohol beyond "just a few sips" in the past month.[136]

We must be sad at each tragedy, but we must also understand that encouraging moderate drinking actually is guilty of contributing to this carnage and actually encourages the alcohol industry. In fact, we believe that Christian leaders who piously call for drinking in moderation are accomplices to the alcohol industry, all the while setting the stage for many more such tragedies. We cannot expect better from the world, but we should expect better from those who claim belief in Christ.

Sadly, all too often, there is in our churches a pervasive silence on these problems and what the Bible says about *wine*. Any subject addressed so frequently in the Bible, such as the dangers of alcohol consumption, deserves mention and study.

And here we must add that that it *is* being seriously studied in the Scientific and Medical world. An article produced by WebMD entitled, "How Alcohol Affects Your Body," states this as its first danger:[137]

> Thirty seconds after your first sip, alcohol races into your brain. It slows down the chemicals and pathways that your brain cells use to send messages. That alters your mood, slows your reflexes, and throws off your balance. You also can't think straight, which you may not recall later, because you'll struggle to store things in long-term memory.

The article goes on to list these effects on the body:

Your Brain Shrinks
Does It Help You Sleep?
More Stomach Acid
Diarrhea and Heartburn
Why You Have to Pee .Again
The Steps to Liver Disease
Pancreas Damage and Diabetes
An Offbeat Heart
A Change in Body Temperature
A Weaker Immune System
Hormone Havoc
Hearing Loss
Thin Bones, Less Muscle

The description of each one of these in the article is down-right scary and certainly is a good reason to practice and to teach abstention.

To add to these effects is the fact that alcohol, even moderately consumed, increases the risk of cancer. It has long been proven that cigarettes kill and the percentage of those in the USA that believe this has risen, which has produced the effect that the number of smokers has dropped "from 46% (1974) to 19% (2014)," according to an article on the web by BMC Public Health.[138] The same article goes on to say:

> There is now robust evidence that low levels of alcohol intake do not provide any protective health benefits, and The WHO International Agency for Research on Cancer (IARC), World Cancer Research Fund and American Institute for Cancer Research have all stated that no level of alcohol consumption is completely safe.

Even if Christians disagree about the meaning of the word "wine" in the Bible, they should be willing to consider the dangers of alcohol. At least Charles Spurgeon, though he personally believed that drinking alcoholic beverages moderately was permitted for Christians and for himself, gave it up in order not to be a stumbling block. When we realize the terrible danger of parents teaching their children that drinking alcohol is blessed by God, it would seem that such parents should consider changing their lifestyle to protect their children. In Romans 14, the apostle Paul discussed the principle of a "strong" brother giving up what he considered to be permissible (eating meat sacrificed to idols), in order not to cause the fall of someone who thought that this would be wrong. He also said in 1 Corinthians 8:13: "Wherefore, if meat make my brother to offend, I will eat no flesh while the world standeth, lest I make my brother to offend."

Peter Masters wrote a book, "Should Christians Drink?" His answer is a resounding "no"! He states:

> We should shudder that the world has taken alcohol and made it such a force for destruction, misery and horror.
>
> We should shudder at the way it subdues the higher senses even of the countless men and women who drink only moderately.
>
> We should shudder away from a product which causes an estimated 10 to 16 million children under eighteen to have to grow up in the living nightmare of a shattered alcoholic home.
>
> We should shudder that the greatest component of the human frame-the rational faculty-is regularly blurred and distorted by alcohol, so that the baser part of the human nature is released.[139]

If we disagree with Masters and with the thesis of this book, we need to go beyond holding tenaciously to what one believes, that drinking moderately is permitted in Scripture, and accept the fact that being willing to give up what one believes to be right for the sake of others and even our own bodies is the right thing to do.

The *evidences* presented in this book that grape juice is present in the Bible and that God never blesses the consumption of alcohol cannot be ignored. This evidence must be presented to give Christians confidence that God does not condone the drinking of alcoholic beverages in any form. Pastors and Bible scholars must fearlessly teach on this subject. Paul said, "Wherefore I take you to record this day, that I am pure from the blood of all men. For I have not shunned to declare unto you all the counsel of God" (Acts 20:26, 27)

CONCLUSION

This book is the result of my search for the truth concerning the presence of grape juice in the Bible. Certain experiences in my life and regular Bible reading made me question that which was current teaching on the subject. When I realized that my acquired belief (that grape juice could not be preserved fresh in Bible times) was wrong and that there were many proofs of the presence of grape juice in the Bible, I felt constrained to write this book to help other Christians know the truth and take a stand against alcohol.

To present these proofs, we made this study follow the same logic as my own studies. We had to consider the challenge that God never contradicts Himself, but only *seems to* be inconsistent or to contradict Himself in His usage of the word "wine" in Scripture.

We saw first, that God blessed Israel and their "wine." He said, "And he will love thee, and bless thee, and multiply thee: he will also bless the fruit of thy womb, and the fruit of thy land, thy corn, and thy wine and thine oil..." (Deut. 7:13). This promise was kept according to 1 Kings 4:25: "And Judah and Israel dwelt safely, every man under his vine and under his fig tree, from Dan even to Beersheba, all the days of Solomon." In the Bible, nothing pictured God's blessing better than the vine. He created it to produce healthy grape juice; He promised it, planned for it, and provided it in the promised land to give His people gladness of heart (Ps. 104:14, 15).

And yet, God also said about "wine" in the Bible: "Woe unto them that rise up early in the morning, that they may follow strong drink; that continue until night, till wine inflames them" (Is. 5:11). A little further, Isaiah says: "Woe unto them that are mighty to drink wine..." (v. 22). These verses show that there were people in Israel who drank "wine" made from the vine and that God condemned this act. God not only condemned drinking "wine," but He promised judgment to Israel for misusing the fruit of the vine. Hosea says (7:1-13):

> The iniquity of Ephraim is discovered, and the wickedness of Samaria, for they commit falsehood;(v. 1)... They make the king glad with their wickedness, and the princes with their lies (v.3).... In the day of our king the princes have made him sick with bottles of wine; he stretched out his hand with mockers (v.5).

Being "sick with wine" is an important transgression!

Next, we continued our study with the meaning of the word wine in Scripture. We determined that there are several Hebrew words used in the Hebrew Old Testament for the product of the vine and for other beverages. These words were translated by one Greek word oinos in the Greek translation of the Old Testament (the LXX) and by one English word wine in the English translations. Because of this, we can conclude that, in Greek and in English, the word used is generic (not specific). The assumption that the word is specifically and uniquely alcoholic wine has led to the present confusion about God's blessing and condemnation of the same product. Studying the Hebrew words helps clear up this confusion. Even with just the English translation, God has been very consistent in giving enough background and context in each use of the word "wine" to permit us to understand why He sometimes blesses the fruit of the vine and at other times curses the use of harmful alcoholic wine. I believe His condemnation and warning against the product have everything to do with when it has been tainted with what causes intoxication (leaven, and thus alcoholic wine). In contrast, I believe His blessing and encouragement have everything to do with the proper use of the product when it is kept unadulterated and used in a way that poses no risk of rendering someone less sober (grape juice). Therefore, we can say that, depending on the context, often the same word in English is used for what amounts to be two very different substances: alcoholic beverages and unfermented grape juice.

To give us a better perspective on the problem, we also studied the historical development of Christian attitudes toward alcohol in our country by briefly looking at the Temperance Movement in Chapter VII.

We continued our search for the truth by going deeper into the study of just how important truth is to God, and how necessary it is for us to understand it as it comes from Him. This led us to a consideration of the necessity of *"rightly dividing"* or interpreting God's Word. We found that proper, historical methods of interpretation are absolutely essential to a proper understanding of biblical truth.

Applying these methods helped us conclude that the Bible does indeed speak much of grape juice. Also, the application of these methods helped us answer the question: Did Jesus make and drink alcoholic wine? Our conclusion was clear-Jesus, the creator of the universe and the Holy Son of God, did not make an alcoholic beverage and give it to those who had already "well drunk." He obeyed God's laws unfailingly and from water created refreshingly delicious grape juice for His friends. Jesus, God's perfect sacrifice for sin, did not drink an alcoholic beverage during the Passover Supper. He fulfilled all of God's qualifications for a perfect sacrifice. He partook only of products that had no leaven in them: unleavened bread and unfermented juice, "the fruit of the vine." This point is very important because it removes the primary excuse that Christians use to permit them to consume alcoholic beverages.

Al and Alice Lunden make a bold statement in their book, *Jesus, the Winemaker, Satan's Most Effective Lie*:

> This book is an expose of an obvious hoax about Christianity's use of wine and other drugs, which has been going on in many Judeo-Christian Churches, and apparently also within Judaism for about seventeen hundred years.

> This hoax, from the church of my youth and through my high school years, regarding the false portrayal of Jesus as being a maker of wine at the Cana wedding, and being a user of wine for Holy Communion at the Last Supper, was directly and largely responsible for my use and abuse of wine and other alcoholic drugs from age twenty-five to age fifty.[140]

The fact of grape juice in the Bible allows us to recognize and affirm that God is consistent in Himself and in His Word. We can state with confidence that He blesses the fruit of the vine, grape juice, and He condemns the use of alcoholic wine. At last, it can be said that God blessed Israel and their grape juice when He said in Deut. 7:13:

> And he will love thee, and bless thee, and multiply thee: he will also bless the fruit of thy womb, and the fruit of thy land, thy corn, and thy grape juice, and thine oil, the increase of thy kine, and the flocks of thy sheep, in the land which he sware unto thy fathers to give thee."

He also said in Isaiah 55:1: "Ho, everyone that thirsteth, come ye to the waters, and he that hath no money; come ye, buy, and eat; yea, come, buy grape juice and milk without money and without price."

We can also state with authority that God condemned the use of alcoholic wine when He said, "Woe unto them that rise up early in the morning, that they may follow strong drink; that continue until night, till (alcoholic) wine inflame them" (Isa. 5:11) and later in the same chapter, "Woe unto them that are mighty to drink (alcoholic) wine…" (Isa. 5:22).

Thus, we arrive at this necessary conclusion: there are two wines in the Bible:

1. In the Bible, God repeatedly blesses and encourages the use of grape juice, which is often translated by "wine" in our English Bibles.
2. In the Bible, God repeatedly condemns the use of alcoholic wine in the strongest terms.
3. Modern Christians should not drink alcoholic beverages-even moderately.

Refusing to believe the presence of grape juice in Scripture is to admit that Christians today have every right to drink alcohol moderately. However, our study in Chapters XI and XII has proved that there is a growing problem with alcohol and that diluting wine or drinking moderately is not the answer. To say that God can bless and curse the same product, depending only on how much one partakes of the product, subtly and gravely implies that God condones or even encourages "playing with fire." To the contrary! God condemns even approaching a product that leads to saying perverse things (Prov. 23:31-33), because it opens the way to temptation. This condemnation is the only act that would be consistent with God's thrice holy and good nature.

Those who would accept the wrong interpretation of Scripture (that God blesses alcoholic beverages) have grossly misunderstood Him. A bad interpretation of Scripture regarding wine will ultimately lead to maligning God's character-a very serious offense! A Christian should never accept an understanding of God's Word that makes God contradict Himself. This is the real issue: God cannot contradict Himself.

Let us accept that God always speaks clearly and truly about what He expects His creatures to do. He tells us specifically in Titus 2:12 that He wants us "to live soberly, righteously, and godly in this present world..." As believers, we are called "the salt of the earth" (Matt. 5:13). Far from shying away from the subject of grape juice and wine in the Bible, we ought to address the subject with confidence and boldness. We who believe God's Word must be eager to see, understand, and share with others what He says in His Word, for God speaks clearly:

> Love not the world, neither the things that are in the world. If any man love the world, the love of the Father is not in him. (1 John 2:15)

> The Lord gave the word: great was the company of those that published it. (Ps. 68:1)

APPENDIX: IS MODERATE DRINKING REALLY SAFE DRINKING?

MA Department of Public Health[141]

Adults are advised to be cautious when consuming alcohol and consider their personal situation before deciding to drink. Contacting your health care provider before changing drinking patterns can help to prevent problems. Remember that a healthy diet, avoidance of smoking, and maintenance of an appropriate level of physical activity and weight can help to maintain a strong heart, as well as enhance one's outlook.

Recent reports

The Bureau of Substance Abuse Services cautions Massachusetts residents to consider their personal circumstance as well as the potential for negative effects before consuming alcohol.

Studies may show that "light or moderate drinkers have lower rates of coronary heart disease than abstainers." Yet this doesn't tell the whole story.[142]

Facts to consider

- Factors such as a healthy diet, physical activity, avoidance of smoking, and maintenance of a healthy weight will help to reduce the risk of heart disease.

- An Addiction Specialist and Senior Scientist at the Centre for Addiction and Mental Health at the University of Toronto states that "the health benefits of alcohol use are generally overstated and are virtually nonexistent for young people. Even small amounts of alcohol increase the risk of injury and boost the chances of developing about sixty diseases."[143]
- The World Health Organization suggests that when differences relating to the individual's social and economic position are corrected, the seeming cardio-protective effects may no longer be found.[144]
- The most recent studies do not necessarily account for crucial, personal differences which greatly affect how alcohol reacts to the body. (See Personal Factors below.)
- Adults should talk to their health care providers before changing their drinking habits.

WHAT PERSONAL FACTORS CONTRIBUTE TO REACTIONS WITH ALCOHOL?

Gender - Moderate drinking levels differ for men and women. This is because women's bodies process alcohol differently, and they are more sensitive to alcohol use.[145]

Age - There are no safe limits of alcohol use for youth or adolescents. Consumption of alcohol under the age of twenty-one is illegal. Older adults, in addition, are much more sensitive to alcohol intake.[146]

Personal and Family History - People with a personal or family history of alcohol problems or alcoholism must be especially cautious as they may not be able to drink alcohol safely.

Medication Intake - Alcohol can interact with some prescription and over-the-counter medication. It is essential to ask individual health care providers before changing drinking patterns.[147]

Pregnancy - Alcohol consumption during pregnancy can seriously affect the mental and physical development of the unborn baby. According to the Health and Nutrition Newsletter of Tufts University, alcoholic beverages should not be consumed by women of childbearing age who may become pregnant or pregnant and lactating women.[148]

WHAT IS "MODERATE DRINKING"?

- According to the World Health Organization, "there may be some danger that talking about a 'safe limit' (for alcohol use) will encourage more of the population to drink and spur light drinkers to drink up to the stated limit."[149]
- Moderate drinking levels are generally defined as no more than one drink per day for women (under age 65) and no more than two drinks per day for men (under 65). These limits are based on differences between the sexes in both weight and metabolism.[150]
- Elderly (above age 65) should limit alcohol intake because their bodies process alcohol differently. The maximum limits of drinks a day for men over 65 is 1 drink per day, and for women over 65 is less than one per day.[151]
- There are no safe limits for alcohol use by youth.
- People with certain diseases, or who are taking over-the-counter or prescription medication should check with their pharmacist or health care provider, as even low levels of alcohol use may cause a reaction.

The personal factors listed above can change the effects of even moderate levels of alcohol use.

WHAT ARE POTENTIAL CONSEQUENCES OF ALCOHOL USE?

Health related problems:[152]

- liver cirrhosis,
- elevated blood pressure,
- variety of types of cancer,
- stroke, and
- damage to unborn children.

Social, legal and safety issues:

- increased risk of family, work, and other problems,
- negative behavior modeling (parents setting examples for youth),
- absenteeism, low productivity,
- financial hardship,
- criminal behavior,
- violence and/or accidental death, and
- driving under the influence of alcohol.

Society at large:

- In addition to the potential individual consequences of increased alcohol consumption, the public may suffer from the promotion of moderate drinking.[153]

- Although drinking is a personal act and an individual responsibility, it is also behavior shaped by our societies and something for which society as a whole has responsibility.[154]

According to the World Health Organization, "measures that influence drinkers in general will also have an impact on heavier drinkers. Promoting increased levels of moderate drinking may in turn increase overall consumption, even for those who should not do so."[155]

SELECT BIBLIOGRAPHY: BOOKS AND ARTICLES PRESENTING "2 WINES" IN THE BIBLE

Bacchiocchi, Samuele. *Wine in the Bible: A Biblical Study on the Use of Alcoholic Beverages*. Berrien Springs, MI: Biblical Perspectives, 1989.

Brumbelow, David R. *Ancient Wine & the Bible: The Case for Abstinence*. Carrollton, GE: Free Church Press, 2011.

Clarke, Adam. *Adam Clarke Commentary*, *Genesis 40:11*. New York: J. Emory and B. Waugh, 1831.

Field, Leon C. Oinos: *A Discussion of the Bible Wine Question*. New York: Phillips & Hunt. 1883. Harvard College Library, digitalized by Google. http://books.google.com/books.

Josephus, *Antiquities of the Jews*, Book 2, Chapter 5, A.D. 94, Kindle Books.

Kirton, John W. *The Water Drinkers of the Bible*. Edinburgh: Lorimer and Gillies, 1885. Harvard University Library digitalized by Google. http://books.google.com/books.

Lumpkins, Peter. *Alcohol Today: Abstinence in an age of Indulgence*. Hannibal Books: Garland Texas, 2009.

Lunden, Al and Alice. *Jesus the Winemaker Satan's Most Effective Lie*. Bloomington, IN: Westbow Press, 2011.

Marshall, George, *The "Strong Drink" Delusion, with its Criminal and Ruinous Results Exposed*. Halifax: The Journal Office, 1855.

This book has been republished by "Forgotten Books," www. Forgotten Books.com.

McGuiggan, Jim. *The Bible, the Saint, and the Liquor Industry.* Lubbock, TX: International Biblical Resources Inc, 1977.

Nott, Eliphalet. *Lectures on Temperance*, New York: Sheldon, Blakeman & Co., 115 Nassau Street, 1857.

Patton, William. *The Laws of Fermentation and the Wines of the Ancients.* New York: National Temperance Society and Publishing House, 1871.

Reynolds. Stephen M., *The Biblical Approach to Alcohol*. Glenside, PA: Lorine L. Reynolds Foundation. 2003.

Teachout, Raymond L. *Adrift from the Gospel.* (Chateau-Richer, Quebec: EBPA, 2011), p. 149.

Teachout, Robert. *Wine the Biblical Imperative: Total Abstinence.* Detroit, MI: Published by Author, 1983.

Van Impe, Jack. *Alcohol, the Beloved Enemy*. Nashville: Thomas Nelson Publishers, 1980.

OTHER BOOKS AND ARTICLES:

Emmons, "His Word is Truth," *Israel My Glory*, Jan/Feb 2009.

Denise, George. *Planting Trust, Knowing Peace*, Grand Rapids: Zondervan, 2005.

Gibson, Caitlin. *The 'sober-curious' movement challenges 'wine mom' culture*, Grand Rapids Press, August 11, 2019.

Geisler, Norman. *Explaining Hermeneutics: A Commentary on the Chicago Statement on Biblical Hermeneutics.* Bastion Books, Matthews, NC: 1983. Kindle Edition.

Geisler, N. L., and Nix, W. E. (1996). *A General Introduction to the Bible* (revised and expanded). Chicago: Moody Press. 1986.

Hobson, Richmond Pearson. *Alcohol and the Human Race.* (Published by Google Books), 1919.

Jaeggli, Randy. *Alcohol and the Human Race: The Christian and Drinking, a Biblical Perspective on Moderation and Abstinence.* Greenville, SC: BJU Press. 2008. This book has been withdrawn from publication.

Josephus. *Antiquities of the Jews*, Book 2, Chapter 5.

Manser, Martin, et al. *The Complete Topical Guide to the Bible.* Grand Rapids, Baker Books, 2017, Kindle Edition.

Milner, Duncan C. *Lincoln and Liquor.* 440 Fourth Avenue, New York: The Neale Publishing Company, 1920.

Peck, Garrett. *The Prohibition Hangover: Alcohol in America from Demon Rum to Cult Cabernet.* Kindle Edition.

Peck, Garrett. *Winemaking in Ancient Israel.* Kindle Edition. Puett, Terry. *A Categorical, Alphabetical Bible Study*, Vol. 2. Pueblo, CO: T&L Publications, 2014, https://books.google.com/ books/ about/A_Categorical_Alphabetical_Bible_Study_V.html?id=v7aUBgAAQBAJ, (accessed 03/05/2019).

Ramm, Bernard. *Protestant Biblical Interpretation.* Grand Rapids: Baker Books, 1970.

Reinstadler, Kym. "'Thou Shalt Not' Revoked." The Grand Rapids Press. Nov. 21, 2009.

Rosen, Maggie. *Drink to This. Health Science Boston Globe.* April 6, 2004.

Stott, John. *Evangelical Truth*. Downers Grove, IL: InterVarsity Press, 1999, pp. 116-117.

Thompson, Robert Ellis. *The Hand of God in American History*. New York: Thomas Crowell & Co, 1902.

ARTICLES ON INTERNET

Baker, R. A. "Wine in the Ancient World." http://www.church history101. com/feedback/wine-ancient-world.php, (accessed 03/18/2019).

Beecher, Lyman. *Six Sermons on Intemperance.* http://utc.iath. virginia.edu/sentiment/sneslbat.html, (accessed 2/25/2019).

Brennan, Tom. "Ignorance Is Bliss." https://concerningjesus.blog spot. com/2015/07/alcohol-9-ignorance-is-bliss.html?m=0, (accessed 03/25/2019).

Chard, Phillip. "Alcohol causes more harm than many less legal substances." https://www.jsonline.com/story/life/green-sheet/advice/ philip-chard/2018/10/12/alcohol-causes-more-harm-than-many-less-legal-substances/1568041002/, (accessed 2/19/2019).

Creech, Mark H. *Prohibition and the legalization of drugs.* http:// www.renewamerica.com/columns/creech/051122, (accessed 3/20/2019).

Driscoll, Mark. *The Radical Reformission.* Zondervan, 1970. Kindle.

Emmons, Richard. "His Word is Truth," *Israel. My Glory, Jan/ Feb 2009* https://israelmyglory.org/article/his-word-is-truth/ hilite=%27 His%27%2C%27Word%27%2C%27Truth%27 (accessed 2/28/2019).

Foster, Susan E., et al. "Alcohol Consumption and Expenditures for Underage Drinking and Adult Excessive Drinking." https://jama-network.com/journals/ jamapediatrics/fullarticle/204917, (accessed 2/7/2019).

Foster, Susan E., Vaughan, Roger D., Foster, William H. "Estimate of the Commercial Value of Underage Drinking and Adult Abusive and Dependent Drinking to the Alcohol Industry," https://jamanet work.com/journals/jamapediatrics/fullarticle/204917?resultClick=, (accessed 2/7/2019).

Geisler, Norman L. "A Christian Perspective on Wine-Drinking." Bibliotheca Sacra: BSAC 139:553 (Jan. 1982). https://www.galaxie.com/article/bsac139-553-04, (accessed 03/22/2019).

Gowin, Joshua. "Your Brain on Alcohol: Is the Conventional Wisdom Wrong about Booze?" https://www.psychologytoday.com /us/blog/you-illuminated/201006/your-brain-alcohol, (accessed 10/05/2018).

Jaret, Peter. "Wine or Welch's? Grape Juice Provides Health Benefits Without Alcohol." http://edition.cnn.com/2000/ HEALTH/alternative /03/31/wine.heart.wmd/, (accessed 3/18/2019).

Kelland, Kate. "Drug Experts Say Alcohol Worse Than Crack or Heroin." *Reuters*. https://www.reuters.com/article/us-drugs-alcohol/drug-experts-say-alcohol-worse-than-crack-or-heroin-idUSTRE6A00O020101101, (accessed 2/7/2019).

Kulikovsky, Andrew S. "Inspiration, Authority and Interpretation." http://www.kulikovskyonline.net/hermeneutics/inspirat.htm, (accessed 3/5/2019).

Marshall. George. *Personal Narratives with Reflections and Remarks.* Halifax, N.S. T Chamberlain, 176 Argyle St. 1866, Harvard College, Google e-books.

May, Ashley. "Alcohol Is a Leading Cause of Death, Disease Worldwide." https://www.usatoday.com/story/news/nation-now/ 2018/08/24/alcohol-death-disease-study-beer-wine/1082443002/, (accessed 2//19/2019).

Miller, Dave. "The Bible Is Its Own Best Interpreter." https://apologetics press.org/apcontent.aspx?category=11& article=1242, (accessed 2/28/2019).

Miller, Norm. Posted on Mar. 20, 2007 http://www.bpnews. net/bpfirstperson.asp?id=25221, (accessed 6/23/2011). Møller, Lars. "How can I drink alcohol safely?" *World Health Organization. Europe.* http://www.euro.who.int/en/health-topics/disease-prevention/alcohol-use/data-and-statistics/q-and-a-how-can-i-drink-alcohol-safely, (accessed 3/20/2019).

Myers, Kim. "5 Stages of the Wine Making Process." http://laurelgray.com/5-stages-wine-making-process, (accessed 3/15/2019).

Nebehay, Stephanie. "Alcohol Kills More than AIDS, TB or Violence: WHO." https:// www.reuters.com /article/us-alcohol-idUS-TRE71A2FM 20110211, (accessed 2/7/2019).

Nordqvist, Christian. "Alcohol Is Most Harmful Drug, Followed by Heroin And Crack." Medical News Today, https://www.medical news today.com/articles/206300.php, (accessed 2/7/2019).

Nordqvist, Christian. "What is alcohol abuse disorder, and what is the treatment?" Medical News Today, (Last updated Tue 29 May 2018). https://medium.com/@stilettocycle/alcohol-abuse-2171de7184f6, (accessed on 03/20/2019).

Rehn, Jurgen, et al. "Alcohol as Damaging as Tobacco." *Nature. April 8, 2004.* Quoted by MA Department of Public Health. Report reproduced in Appendix.

Reinstadler, Kym. *Alcohol, Acts 29 and the SBC.* The Grand Rapids Press, Nov. 21, 2009, front page, article by Kym Reinstadler, reproduced by permission.

Shelnutt, Kate. "Pour One for the Pastor? Evangelical Perspectives on Alcohol and the Church," Believe it or not. https://blog. chron.com/ believeitornot/2010/07/pour-one-for-the-pastor-evangelical-perspectives-on-alcohol-and-the-church/, (accessed 3/18/2019).

Showers, Renald. "The Foundations of Faith: God Is True and Truth." https://www.foi.org/free_resource/foundations-faith-god-true-and-truth, (accessed 2/28/2019).

Shrader, Rick. "Bible Wine." http://aletheiabaptistministries.org/ Blog/august-"bible-wine"/, (accessed 2/7/19).

Soniak, Matt. "Does Drinking Alcohol Kill Brain Cells?" *Big Questions.* http://mentalfloss.com/article/49024/does-drinking-alcohol-kill-brain-cells (accessed 3/10/19).

Stein, Robert H. "Wine-Drinking In New Testament Times." *The Bible's Word on Alcohol.* http://www.searchthescriptures. org/ blog/the-bible-s-word-on-alcohol/print, (accessed 03/18/2019).

Tait, Jennifer L. Woodruff. "Raise a Juice Box to the Temperance Movement." https://www.christianitytoday.com/history/2017/ march/welch-grape juice-history-temperance-movement.html, (accessed 2/7/19).

Tanski, Susanne E., McClure, Auden C., Zhigang, Li. "Cued Recall of Alcohol Advertising on Television and Underage Drinking Behavior." https://jamanetwork.com/journals/jamapediatrics/ full article/2089643?resultClick=1, (accessed 2/7/2019).

Tapert, Susan F. "Alcohol and the Adolescent Brain-Human Studies." *National Institute on Alcohol Abuse and Alcoholism.* https:// pubs.niaaa.nih.gov/publications/arh284/205-212.html, (accessed 4/20/2019)

Thornton, Mark. "Alcohol Prohibition Was a Failure." https://
www.cato. org/policy-analysis/alcohol-prohibition-was-failure,
(accessed 2/25/2019).

"New Scientific Study: No Safe Level of Alcohol." IHME. http://
www. healthdata.org/news-release/new-scientific-study-no-
safe-level-alcohol, (accessed 11/15/2018).

Whetan, D.D. *Methodist Quarterly Review*. New York: Phillips &
Hunt, 1882. Available Google Books.

"A Comparison of Gender-Linked Population Cancer Risks between
Alcohol and Tobacco: How Many Cigarettes Are There in a
Bottle of Wine?" *BMC Public Health*. https://www.ncbi.nlm.
nih.gov/pmc/ articles/PMC6437970, (accessed 04/01/2019).

"Alcohol Statistics." *Alcohol: What do these things have in Common*.
https://slideplayer.com/slide/10380852/, (accessed 2/2/19).

"Alcohol Use Disorder." *Mayo Clinic*. https://www.mayo clinic.org/
diseases-conditions/alcohol-use-disorder/symptoms-causes/
syc-20369243, (accessed 4/20/2019).

"Alcohol and Your Brain." Science NetLinks. http://science netlinks.
com/student-teacher-sheets/alcohol-and-your-brain/,
(accessed 03/21/2019).

"American Temperance Society." Wikileaks. https://en.wiki-pedia.
org/wiki/AmericanTemperanceSociety, (accessed 5/8/2019).

"Alcohol deaths are up 35%-and 67% among women. What's
happening?" https://www.advisory.com/daily-briefing
/2018/11/29/alcohol-deaths

"Context." https://en.oxforddictionaries.com/definition/context,
(accessed 2/28/2019).

"Defrutum." https://ipfs.io/ipfs/QmXoypizjW3WknFiJn KLwHCnL72 vedxjQkDDP1mXWo6uco/wiki/Defrutum.html, (accessed 2/15/2019).

"Education: Going Back to the Booz." http://www.time.com/time /magazine/article/0,9171,912518,00. html#ixzz1QIBrCUjP, (accessed 3/19/2019).

"Evidence from Long-Term Studies." *Alcohol Advertising and Youth.* http://www.camy.org/resources/fact-sheets/alcohol-advertis-ing-and-youth/index.html, (accessed 3/18/2019).

"Excessive Drinking is Draining the US Economy." *CDC Features.* https://www.cdc.gov/features/costsofdrinking/index.html, (accessed 2/7/2019).

Guerzoni Mosto D'Uva "Biodynamic Grape Juice." https://www. amazon.com/ Guerzoni-Mosto-Biodynamic-25-Ounce Bottles/ dp/B001J5T4NO, (accessed 03/27/2019).

"Hermeneutics: The Eight Rules of Biblical Interpretation." *Hermeneutics: How To Interpret The Bible.* http://www.apolo-getics index.org/5846-biblical-interpretation-rules, (accessed 3/14/2019).

"Hermeneutics: 8 Principles: Rule of Definition." https://quizlet. com/ 136610765/hermeneutics-8-principles-flash-cards/, (accessed 04/08/2019).

"How can alcohol be blamed for 100,000 deaths each year?" http:// www.come-over.to/FAS/alcdeath.html, (accessed 2/7/2019).

"Is Moderate Drinking Really Safe Drinking?" *Moderate drinking.* https://www.mass.gov/service-details/moderate-drinking, (accessed 3/20/2019).

"It Led to Prohibition." *American Temperance Society,* https://www.alcoholproblemsandsolutions.org/american-temperance-society-led-prohibition/, (accessed 2/25/2019).

Lincoln and Liquor. The Neale Publishing Company, 440 Fourth Avenue, New York, 1920. https://archive.org/details/lincoln liquor01miln/page/15, (accessed 2/25/2019).

Moderation vs. Total Abstinence, or *Dr. Crosby and His Reviewers.* New York: The National Temperance Society and Publication House, 1881.

"Must." http://en.wikipedia.org/wiki/Must, (accessed 3/15/2019).

Picture is from https://3.bp.blogspot.com /fOXRVCH9ETI/UI8k T5FbHDI/AAAAAAAAA Po/6sxjOIBvuxE/s1600Treading+ wine-press,+tb100806677+800.jpg, (accessed 03/22/12019).

"Review of Dr. Crosby's Calm view of temperance." http://books.google.com/books, (accessed 2/28/2019).

"Scientific Temperance from a German Point of View." *School Physiology Journal,* https://archive.org/details/school physiology10bost/page/12, (accessed 11/16/2019).

"Straight to Your Head," *How Alcohol Affects Your Body* (WebMD). https://www.webmd.com/mental-health/addiction/ss/slideshow-alcohol-body-effects, (accessed 04/01/2019).

The Holy Bible: English Standard Version. 2001 (Lk. 24:21). Wheaton, IL: Standard Bible Society.

"Underage Drinking Statistics." *National Institute on Alcoholic Abuse and Alcoholism.* https://pubs.niaaa.nih.gov/publications/UnderageDrinking/UnderageFact.htm, (Accessed 03/21/2019).

"Understanding Alcohol Use Disorders and Their Treatment." *American Psychological Association.* https://www.apa.-org/ helpcenter/alcohol-disorders, (accessed 8/27/2019

"Welcome to The Amethyst Initiative." *Amethyst Initiative: Rethink the Drinking Age.* http://www.theamethystinitiative.org, (accessed 3/18/2019).

"What is Alcohol Abuse." *Alcohol Abuse.* https://drugabuse.com/ alcohol/, (accessed 03/20/2019).

Wine. http://www.webster-dictionary.org/definition/wine, (accessed 03/27/2019).

Wine in the Ancient World. http://www.churchhistory101.com/ feedback/wine-ancient-world.php, (accessed 02/18/2019).

Woe to the Drinker of Wine. https://islamqa.info/en/answers/ 38145/woe-to-the-drinker-of-wine, (accessed 2/25/2019).

ENDNOTES

1   Gowin, Joshua. *Your Brain on Alcohol: Is the Conventional Wisdom Wrong about Booze?* https://www.psychologytoday. com/us/blog/you-illuminated/201006/your-brain-alcohol, accessed 10/05/2018.

2   "Alcohol deaths are up 35%—and 67% among women. What's happening?" https://www.advisory.com/daily-briefing /2018/11/29/alcohol-deaths, accessed 1/31/2019.

3   Caitland Gibson, Grand Rapids Press, 8/11/2019

4   Ibid

5   The Grand Rapids Press, Nov. 21, 2009, front page, article by Kym Reinstadler, reproduced by permission.

6   Mark Driscoll, *The Radical Reformission.* Zondervan, 1970. Kindle.

7   Kate Kelland, "Drug Experts Say Alcohol Worse Than Crack or Heroin." Reuters. https://www.reuters.com/article/ us-drugs-alcohol/drug-experts-say-alcohol-worse-than-crack-or-heroin-idUSTRE6A000O20101101, accessed 2/7/2019.

8   Christian Nordqvist, "Alcohol Is Most Harmful Drug, Followed By Heroin And Crack," Medical News Today, http://www.med-icalnews today.com /articles/ 206300.php, accessed 2/7/2019.

9   "Experts: Alcohol More Harmful Than Crack or Heroin," WebMD. https://www.webmd.com/mental-health/addic-tion/news/20101101 /alcohol-more-harmful-than-crack-or-heroin#1, accessed 2/7/2019.

10 "How can alcohol be blamed for 100,000 deaths each year?" http://www.come-over.to/FAS/alcdeath.htm, accessed 2/7/2019.

11 Stephanie Nebehay, "Alcohol kills more than AIDS, TB or violence: WHO." Reuters. https://www.reuters.com/article/us-alcohol-idUSTRE71A2FM20110211, accessed 2/7/2019.

12 "Excessive Drinking is Draining the US Economy." CDC Features. https://www.cdc.gov/features/costsofdrinking/index.html, accessed 2/7/2019.

13 Susan Foster, et al. "Alcohol Consumption and Expenditures for Underage Drinking and Adult Excessive Drinking." Jama Pediatrics. https://jamanet work.com/journals/ jamapediatrics/fullarticle/204917, accessed 2/7/2019.

14 "Alcohol Statistics," Alcohol: What do these things have in Common. https://slideplayer.com/slide/10380852/, accessed 2/2/19.

15 Susanne E. Tanski, Auden C. McClure, Li Zhigang. "Cued Recall of Alcohol Advertising on Television and Underage Drinking Behavior." https://jamanetwork.com/journals/jamapediatrics/fullarticle/2089643?resultClick=1, accessed 2/7/2019.

16 Rick Shrader, "Bible Wine." http://aletheiabaptistministries.org/Blog /august-qbible-wineq/, accessed 3/12/2019.

17 CHAPTER NOTES

Jennifer L Woodruff Tait. "Raise a Juice Box to the Temperance Movement," https://www.christianitytoday.com/history/2017/march/welch-grape-juice-history-temperance-movement.html. (Accessed 2/7/19.)

18 George Marshall, "The "Strong Drink" Delusion, with its Criminal and Ruinous Results Exposed." The Journal Office, Halifax, 1855, p. 7. This book has been republished by "Forgotten Books," www.Forgotten Books.com.

19 Leon C. Field, "Oinos: A Discussion of the Bible Wine Question," pp. 84, 85.

20 Eliphalet Nott, Lectures on Temperance, New York: Sheldon, Blakeman & Co.., 115 Nassau Street, 1857, pp. 53, 54.

21 Picture is from https://3.bp.blogspot.com /fOXRV-CH9ETI/ UI8kT5Fb HDI/AAAAAAAAPo/6sxjOIB-vuxE/s1600/ Treading+winepress,+tb100806677+800.jpg, (accessed 3/22/12019).

22 "Must." https://en.wikipedia.org/wiki/Must (Accessed 3/15/2019).

23 Samuel Bacchiocchi, Wine in the Bible: A Biblical Study on the Use of Alcoholic Beverages, Berrien Springs, MI: Biblical Perspectives, 1989, p. 58.

24 R.A. Baker, "Wine and Alcohol in the Bible" by http://www. church history101.com/feedback/wine-ancient-world.php, (accessed 02/18/2019).

25 Robert Teachout, (brother of present author), Wine the Biblical Imperative: Total Abstinence, Detroit: Published by Author, 1983, p. 21.

26 "Wine." http://www.webster-dictionary.org/definition/wine, (accessed 03/27/2019).

27 "Biodynamic Grape Juice." https://www.amazon.com/ Guerzoni-Mosto-Biodynamic-25-Ounce-Bottles/dp/ B001J5T4NO, (accessed 03/27/2019).

28 Robert Teachout, op. cit., pp. 73, 74. He analyses each Hebrew word in the O.T. and shows its meaning, grape juice or wine.

29 Josephus, Antiquities of the Jews, Book 2, Chapter 5.

30 Adam Clarke Commentary, Genesis 40:11, cited by Leighton G. Campbell, "Why true creationists Believe that Jesus did not make alcohol," p. 123.

31 Cited by William Patton, Bible Wines: Or, The Laws of Fermentation and Wines of the Ancients, p.72.

32 Marshall, pp. 22, 23.

33 https://concerningjesus.blogspot.com/2015/07/alcohol-9-ig-norance-is-bliss.html?m=0, (Accessed 03, 25, 2019).

34 Patton, p. 34.

35 Patton, pp. 36, 37.

36 Patton, p. 39.

37 Marshall, p. 23.

38 https://islamqa.info/en/answers/38145/woe-to-the-drinker-of-wine, (accessed 2/25/2019).

39 Pliny, ancient Roman nobleman, scientist and historian, author of, Pliny's Natural History said: Some grapes will last all through the winter if the clusters are hung by a string from the ceiling... Cited by Jim McGuiggan, The Bible, the Saint, & the Liquor Industry, 1977, p.64.

40 Jennifer Tate, op. cit.

41 Field, op. cit., pp. 19-30.

42 Richmond Pearson Hobson, Alcohol and the Human Race, (Published by Google Books). 1919, p. 8

43 "Defrutum," https://ipfs.io/ipfs/QmXoypizjW3Wkn FiJnKLwHCnL 72vedxjQkDDP1mXWo6uco/wiki/Defrutum.html (Accessed 2/15/2019).

44 Patton, p. 92.

45 Phillip Chard. "Alcohol causes more harm than many less legal substances." https://www.jsonline.com/story/life/ green-sheet/advice/philip-chard/2018/10/12/alcohol-caus-es-more-harm-than-many-less-legal-substances/1568041002/, (accessed 2//19/2019).

46 Ashley May. "Alcohol is a leading cause of death, dis-ease worldwide." https://www.usatoday.com/story/news/ nation-now/2018/08/24/alcohol-death-disease-study-beer-wine/1082443002/, accessed 2//19/2019).

47 Stephen M Reynolds. "The Biblical Approach to Alcohol," Glenside, PA: Lorine L. Reynolds Foundation. 2003, pp. 3-16.

48 Dr. Reynold discusses this term, "when it is red" at length in "The Biblical approach to Alcohol," pp. 5-9, coming to the con-clusion that it does not refer to the color of the drink, but to its alcoholic nature.

49 Garrett Peck. The Prohibition Hangover. Kindle Edition.

50 https://www.cato.org/policy-analysis/alcohol-prohibi-tion-was-failure, (Accessed 2/25/2019).

51 Peck, Garrett. Prohibition Hangover. Kindle Edition.

52 Robert Ellis Thompson, "The Hand of God in American History: A Study of National Politics," New York: Thomas Crowell& Co., p. 119.

53 Duncan C. Milner, "Lincoln and Liquor," New York: 440 Fourth Avenue, The Neale Publishing Company, 1920, p. 15.

54 Peter Lumpkins, "Alcohol Today: Abstinence in an age of Indulgence, Garland Texas: Hannibal Books:, 2009, p. 119.

55 David R. Brumbelow, "Ancient Wine and the Bible." Carrolton, GA: Free Church Press, 2011, p. 101.

56 Milton Maxwell, "The Washington Movement." https:// silkworth.net/ pdf/TheWashingtonianMovement_ ReffrenceAndResource.pdf (Accessed

57 Lyman Beecher. "Six Sermons on Intemperance." Boston: T.R. Marvin, 1827, p. 7.

58 "American Temperance Society," Wikileaks. https://en.wi-ki-pedia.org/wiki/AmericanTemperanceSociety (Accessed 5/8/2019).

59 George Marshall, "Personal Narratives with Reflections and Remarks." Halifax: N.S. T Chamberlain, 176 Argyle St 1866, Harvard College, Google e-books, p. 74. (Accessed 04/24/2019).

60 Eliphalet Nott, "Lectures on Temperance" p. 265, 267.

61 "Moderation vs. Total Abstinence or Dr. Crosby and his Reviewers." New York: The National Temperance Society and Publication House, 1881, p. 90.

62 Leon C Field, "Oinos: A Discussion of the Bible Wine Question." NY, NY: Phillips & Hunt, 1883; p.17.

63 Ibid

64 Ibid

65 D.D. Whetan, "Methodist Quarterly Review," New York: Phillips & Hunt, 1882, p. 117. Available Google Books.

66 Review of Dr. Crosby's Calm view of temperance, http://books. google.com/books (Accessed 2/28/2019).

67 Emmons, "His Word is Truth," Israel My Glory, Jan/Feb 2009 https://israelmyglory.org/article/his-word-is-truth/?hi-lite=%27His%27% 2C%27Word%27%2C%27Truth%27,) Accessed 2/28/2019).

68 Renald Showers The Foundations of Faith: God is True and Truth https://www.foi.org/free_resource/foundations-faith-god-true-and-truth. (Accessed 2/28/2019).

69 Raymond L. Teachout, "Adrift from the Gospel," Chateau-Richer, QC: EBPA, 2011, p. 148.

70 His quote from Stott is from John Stott, "Evangelical Truth" (Downers Grove, IL.: InterVarsity Press, 1999), pp. 116-117.

71 Raymond L. Teachout, ibid, pp. 116-117.

72 The material under the headings A, B, and C are taken directly from Teachout, Raymond L., "Adrift from the Gospel", EBPA, pages 224-227 with the permission of the author. It is reproduced without italics.

73 Cited by Reynald Showers: https://www.foi.org/free_resource/foundations-faith-god-true-and-truth/ (Accessed 2/28/2019).

74 Miller, Dave. "The Bible is its Own Best Interpreter." https://apologetics press.org/apcontent.aspx?category=11&article=1242, (accessed 2/28/2019).

75 The Holy Bible: English Standard Version. 2001 (Lk. 24:21). Wheaton: Standard Bible Society.

76 "Context." https://en.oxforddictionaries.com/definition/context, (accessed 2/28/2019). http://www.apologeticsindex.org/5846-biblical-interpretation-rules, (accessed 3/14/2019)

77 "Hermeneutics: The Eight Rules of Biblical Interpretation," Hermeneutics: How To Interpret The Bible. http://www.apologeticsindex.org/5846-biblical-interpretation-rules, (accessed 3/14/2019).

78 Bernard Ramm, "Protestant Biblical Interpretation," Grand Rapids, Baker Books, p. 13.

79 Andrew S. Kulikovsky, "Inspiration, Authority and Interpretation." http://www.kulikovskyonline.net/hermeneutics/inspirat.htm (Accessed 3/5/2019).

80 Terry Puett, "A Categorical, Alphabetical Bible Study Vol. 2." Pueblo, CO: T&L Publications, p. 508, https://books.google.com/ books/about/A_Categorical_Alphabetical_Bible_Study_V.html?id=v7aUBgAAQBAJ. (Accessed 03/05/2019).

81 Geisler, N. L., & Nix, W. E. (1996). A General Introduction to the Bible (revised and expanded.) (76–77). Chicago: Moody Press, p. 74.

82 George, Denise. Planting trust, Knowing Peace, Grand Rapids, Zondervan, p. 161.

83 Manser, Martin, et al. "The Complete Topical Guide to the Bible," Grand Rapids, Baker Books, 2017, Kindle Edition. Winemaker.

84 David Brumbelow, Ibid, pp. 177,178. He cites Jerome (AD 400) and G.W. Samson.

85 "Hermeneutics: 8 Principles: Rule of Definition." https://quizlet.com/ 136610765/hermeneutics-8-principles-flash-cards/. (accessed 04/08/2019).

86 Puett, p. 508.

87 Summit I of the International Council on Biblical Inerrancy took place in Chicago on October 26-28, 1978 for the purpose of affirming afresh the doctrine of the inerrancy of Scripture. Norman Geisler, R. C. Sproul. "Explaining Hermeneutics: A Commentary on the Chicago Statement on Biblical Hermeneutics." Matthews, NC: Bastion Books, 1983. Kindle Edition.

88 The Pulpit Commentary: Exodus (Vol. 1), Ex. 11.10.

89 Kim Myers, "5 Stages Of The Wine Making Process." http:// laurel gray.com/5-stages-wine-making-process, (accessed 3/15/2019).

90 Peter Lumpkins, op. cit., p. 141.

91 Part of the results of which are found on pages 21 and 33 of this book.

92 Norman Geisler L, "A Christian Perspective on Wine Drinking." Bibliotheca Sacra: BSAC 139:553 (Jan. 1982). https://www.galaxie.com/article/bsac139-553-04, (accessed 03/220/2019), (accessed 03/22/2019).

93 Etymology is the study of the history of words, their origins, and how their form and meaning have changed over time. Garrett Peck, Winemaking in Ancient Israel. Kindle Edition.

94 Robert H. Stein, "Wine-Drinking in New Testament Times," The Bible's Word on Alcohol. http://www.searchthescriptures.org/blog/the-bible-s-word-on-alcohol/print, (accessed (03/18/22019).

95 Garrett Peck, Ibid.

96 R. A. Baker, "Wine in the Ancient World," http://www.com/feedback/ wine-ancient-world.php, (accessed 03/18/2019).

97 Ibid.

98 George Marshall, op. cit., p. 15.

99 Nott, Eliphalet, Lectures on Biblical Temperance (Turner & Co., London: 1963), p. 68. (Available from Google Books.)

100 Ibid, p. 45

101 Ibid, p. 53

102 Van Impe, J., Alcohol The Beloved Enemy (Nashville: Thomas Nelson Publishers, 1980), p. 7.

103 Lumpkins, op. cit., p. 119.

104 Ibid, p.31.

105 http://www.renewamerica.com/columns/creech/051122, (accessed 3/20/2019).

106 https://www.christianpost.com/news/prohibition-and-the-legalization-of-drugs.html, (accessed 4/4/2019).

107 http://www.time.com/time/magazine/article/0,9171,912518,00.html#ixzz1QIBrCUjP, (accessed 3/19/2019).

108   Van Impe, Jack, op. cit. p. 19.

109   Robert Jaeggli, Christian and Drinking, a Biblical Perspective on Moderation and Abstinence (Greenville, SC: BJU Press, 2008), p. 4.

110   http://www.camy.org/resources/fact-sheets/alcohol-advertising-and-youth/index.html (accessed 3/18/2019).

111   http://www.theamethystinitiative.org, (accessed 3/18/2019).

112   http://www.amethystinitiative.org/statement/, (accessed 3/18/2019).

113   Lumpkins, op. cit.., p. 21.

114   Lumpkins, op. cit., p. 31.

115   Lumpkins, op cit., pp. 19-35.

116   Eliphalet Nott, "Lectures on Temperance," p. 318.

117   Rehn, Jurgen, et al. "Alcohol as Damaging as Tobacco." Nature. April 8, 2004. Quoted by MA Department of Public Health. Report reproduced in Appendix.

118   Peter Jaret, "Wine or Welch's? Grape juice provides health benefits without alcohol." http://edition.cnn.com/2000/HEALTH/alternative /03/31/wine.heart.wmd/, (accessed 3/18/2019).

119   "Scientific Temperance from a German Point of View." School Physiology Journal. https://archive.org/details/school physiology10bost/page/12, (accessed 11/16/2019).

120   "Alcohol use disorder" Mayo Clinic. https://www.mayo clinic.org/ diseases-conditions/alcohol-use-disorder/ symptoms-causes/syc-20369243, (accessed 4/20/2019).

121   https://pubs.niaaa.nih.gov/publications/arh284/205-212. htm, (accessed 4/20/2019)

122   http://mentalfloss.com/article/49024/does-drinking-alcohol-kill-brain-cells (accessed 3/10/19).

123   http://www.euro.who.int/en/health-topics/disease-prevention/alcohol-use/data-and-statistics/q-and-a-how-can-i-drink-alcohol-safely, (accessed 3/20/2019).

124   https://www.psychologytoday.com/us/blog/you-illuminated/201006/your-brain-alcohol, (accessed 10/05/2018).

125   See Appendix.

126   Lumpkins, op. cit., p. 81.

127   https://blog.chron.com/believeitornot/2010/07/pour-one-for-the-pastor-evangelical-perspectives-on-alcohol-and-the-church/, (accessed 3/18/2019).

128   Field, p, 11.

129   http://sciencenetlinks.com/student-teacher-sheets/alcohol-and-your-brain/, (accessed 03/21/2019).

130   McGuiggan, Jim. The Bible, the Saint, & the Liquor Industry. (Lubbock, TX: International Biblical Resources, Inc., 1977), p. 23.

131   https://drugabuse.com/alcohol/, (accessed 03/20/2019).

132   Understanding Alcohol Use Disorders and Their Treatment https://www.apa.org/helpcenter/alcohol-disorders, (accessed 8/27/2019

133   https://drugabuse.com/library/alcoholism/, (accessed 03/20/2019).

134   https://medium.com/@stilettocycle/alcohol-abuse-2171de7184f6, (accessed on 03/20/2019).

135   Susan F. Tapert. "Alcohol and the Adolescent Brain-Human Studies," National Institute on Alcohol Abuse and Alcoholism. https://pubs.niaaa.nih.gov/publications/arh284/205-212.htm, (accessed 4/20/2019).

136   Ibid.

137   https://www.webmd.com/mental-health/addiction/ss/slideshow-alcohol-body-effects, (accessed 04/01/2019).

138   A comparison of gender-linked population cancer risks between alcohol and tobacco: how many cigarettes are there in a bottle of wine?" BMC Public Health. https://www.ncbi.nlm.nih.gov/pmc/ articles/PMC6437970, (accessed 04/01/2019).

139   Masters, Peter, "Should Christians Drink," Sword & Trowel, (London: Metropolitan Tabernacle), pp. 16, 17.

140   Al and Alice Lunden, Jesus, the Winemaker, Satan's Most Effective Lie, (Bloomington, IN: Westbow Press), p. vii.

141   http://www.mass.gov/Eeohhs2/docs/dph/substance_abuse/prevention_advice_moderate_drinking_safe.pdf, (accessed May 2010).

142   https://www.mass.gov/service-details/moderate-drinking, (accessed 03/26/2019).

143   Rehn, Jurgen, et al. "Alcohol as Damaging as Tobacco." Nature. April 8, 2004.

144   "National Institute on Alcohol Abuse and Alcoholism." Alcohol Alert. No.16 PH 315. April 1992.

145   The World Health Organization. The Issue. Health Evidence Network. 2005.

146   Rehn, Jurgen, et al. "Alcohol as Damaging as Tobacco." Nature. April 8, 2004.

147   Massachusetts Department of Public Health, Bureau of Substance Abuse Services and Bureau of Family and Community Health, The Massachusetts Health Promotion Clearinghouse of The Medical Foundation. Healthy Aging: Medications and Alcohol.

148   Dietary Guidelines for Americans, 2005. Retrieved from: www.health.gov 2/16/05.

149   "National Institute on Alcohol Abuse and Alcoholism." Alcohol Alert. No.16 PH 315. April 1992

150   The World Health Organization. The Issue. Health Evidence Network. 2005.

151   Massachusetts Department of Public Health, Bureau of Substance Abuse Services and Bureau of Family and Community Health, The Massachusetts Health Promotion Clearinghouse of The Medical Foundation. Healthy Aging: Medications and Alcohol.

152   Dietary Guidelines for Americans, 2005. Retrieved from: www.health.gov. 2/16/05

153   Edwards, Griffith. Alcohol policy: securing a positive impact on health. Retrieved from: rom:www.euro.who.int/mediacentre/PressBackgrounders/2001/200110022. 1/26/05.

154   Ibid.

155   National Institute on "Alcohol Abuse and Alcoholism." Alcohol Alert. No.16 PH 315. April 1992.

CPSIA information can be obtained
at www.ICGtesting.com
Printed in the USA
LVHW082300020920
664937LV00005B/88

9 781630 501105